PIGSKIN
PALEO

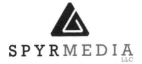

SPYR MEDIA
LLC

PIGSKIN PALEO

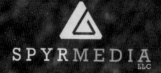

SPYR MEDIA
LLC

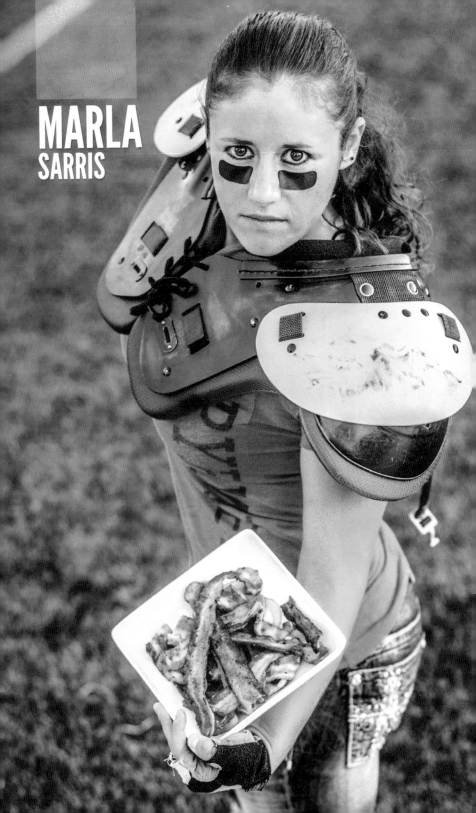

MARLA
SARRIS

Published by Spyr Media, LLC.

ISBN-13: 978-0615693491
ISBN-10: 0615693490

This book is for educational purposes. The publisher and author of this instructional book are not responsible in any manner whatsoever for any adverse effects arising directly or indirectly as a result of the information provided in this book.

Cover photo, cover design and book design by Jeff Sarris.
All photography copyright © Marla Sarris and Jeff Sarris.

First edition.

This book is dedicated to my husband Jeff for all the encouragement, support, time and energy you've given me over the last twelve years. There's no one else I'd rather spend the rest of my life with, doing what I love and sharing memories through travel, business and life. Thank you for all your hard work in getting this book together and also for being my personal taste tester along the way. I love you.

FOREWORD | VIC MAGARY

Modern society whirls by us at an ever increasing pace with every text message, email notification, remote control channel surf, and click of a mouse. But despite the speed of technology and all of the modern conveniences it provides, the human body hasn't changed much in its need for real food.

Prior to the advent of agriculture we did not consume bread or pasta or brightly colored artificially sweetened cereal being marketed with an equally colorful and artificially sweet cartoon character. We ate what we killed or what we foraged from the earth. We hunted and we gathered. If we couldn't eat it raw or cooked with nothing more than a pointy stick and an open flame, then we didn't eat it. And this is the foundation of what is known as the Paleo diet.

The Paleo diet consists of eating lots of vegetables, some meat (to include eggs and seafood), and small amounts of fruit, nuts and seeds. The lines can get blurred sometimes when it comes to potatoes and dairy, but the Paleo diet is not about dogma - it's about eating in a manner for optimum health.

I do not care if this "Paleo diet" is accurate from an anthropological standpoint or not. I only care that in over 10 years of helping people lose weight and get fit, it has been the most effective way of eating for helping my clients reach their health and fitness goals. The only complaint I've ever had from clients has not been the effectiveness of the diet, but that it can at times seem repetitive and boring. And that's where Marla's Pigskin Paleo Cookbook ends all excuses.

This cookbook brings the flavor like no other Paleo cookbook that I've read. Marla's creativity in the kitchen will have your Paleo meals bursting with flavor in a presentation that is also pleasing to the eye whether for an intimate dinner or a party for the next big game. So for the sake of your taste buds and your

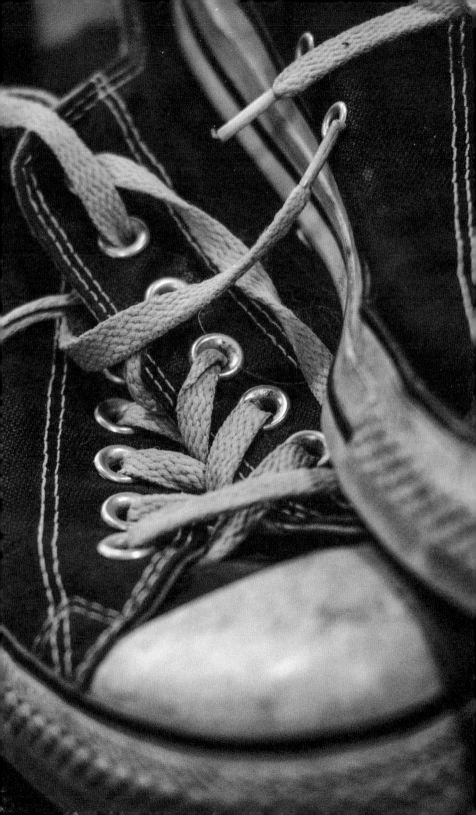

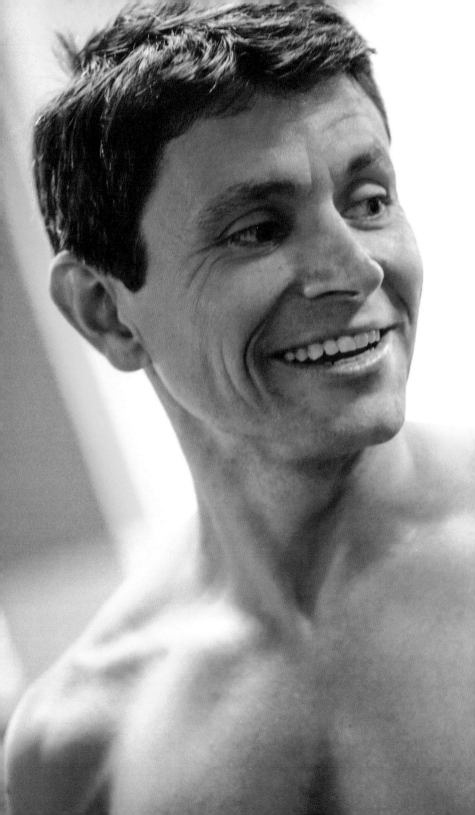

VIC MAGARY is a U.S. Army Infantry veteran and has been helping people lose weight and get fit since 2001. You can learn more about how to take your fitness to the next level without hype or gimmicks at VicMagary.com.

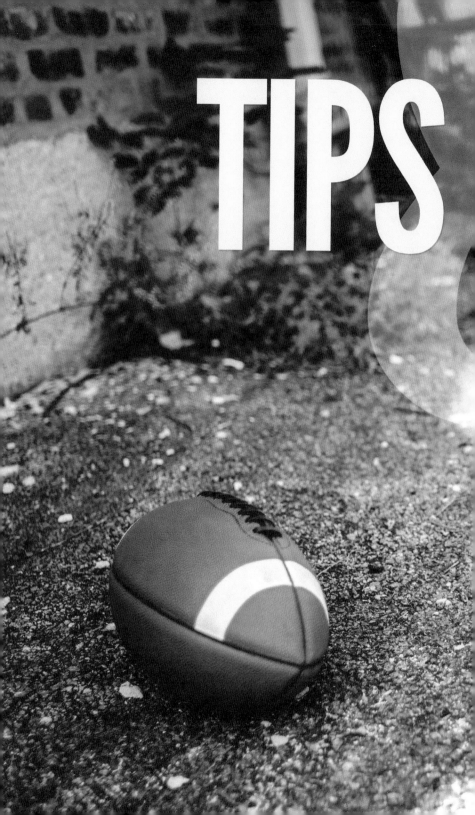

TIPS

TRICKS

Recipes range from **10 MINUTES TO 6 HOURS** because I'm consistent like that

Read the entire recipe to **LEARN FROM MY MISTAKES**

Most recipes use common utensils and ingredients, **YOU DON'T NEED MUCH** to create a tasty meal

Hot pans will burn arms, legs and flying limbs so **TAKE YOUR TIME** *I tend to forget this one* ;)

I constantly fly by the seat of my pants, so don't hesitate to **CHANGE UP THE RECIPES AND HAVE FUN.** Make them your own then be sure to head over to MARLAsarris.com to share your creations!

ABOUT | MARLA SARRIS

Hey there, I'm Marla Sarris and this book is a little extension of me. Three years ago I quit my job as a high school Algebra teacher and decided to focus on figuring out what I really wanted out of life.

At that time me and my husband Jeff embraced minimalism, pairing down to just the necessities. No longer being surrounded by clutter is the catalyst that has allowed us to discover what truly makes us happy.

We've done a lot in the last three years. In no particular order, we've travelled and blogged about our adventures, I spent more time cooking and began to approach meal planning as I did lesson planning, I've made fitness more of a priority in my life, instead of just getting to it when it was convenient, I finally signed up for, and completed, two triathlons, with my current goal being to complete an Olympic distance triathlon next summer, we expanded Jeff's web design and development company by teaming up with Dave LaTulippe and founding Spyr Media and finally we started six4eleven Photography where we shoot people right in the face.

We've been following the Primal/Paleo lifestyle since 2009, but after quitting my job I was able to really dive into the fun of creating in the kitchen and quickly started sharing my results online. After receiving such amazing support from friends, family and the interwebs I decided it was time to create a little something special for everyone.

Thank you so much for picking up Pigskin Paleo. I can't wait to hear what you think!

Enjoy!

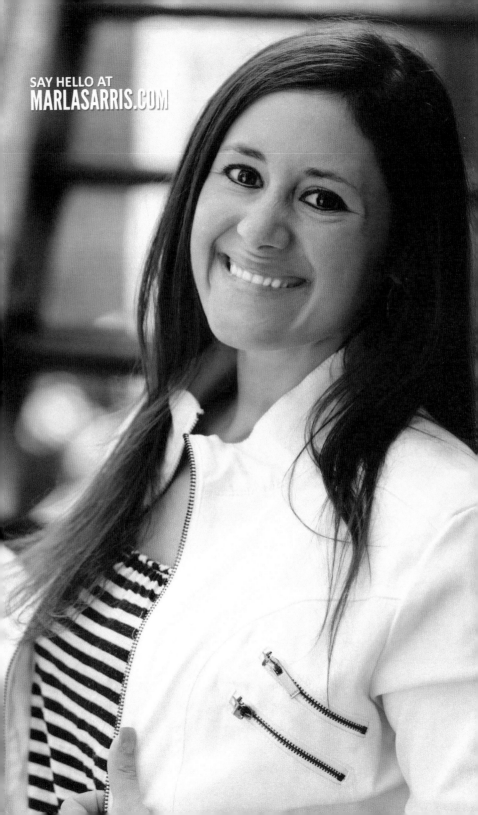

PRE-GAME APPETIZERS

KICKOFF SIDEDISHES

GAMETIME ENTREES

POST-GAME DESSERTS

INTRODUCTION

This book covers some of my favorite go-to meals. Whether I'm preparing food for just my husband and me or for a group of friends who are over to watch the game, these recipes are always crowd pleasers. That said though, what better day for a Paleo feast than gameday, watching with friends? (and ideally a gameday consisting of watching Chicago destroy Green Bay) ;)

No matter the occasion, I love to serve fresh veggies and guacamole, but I also have quite the affinity for bacon. After experimenting for months creating and sharing bacon recipes in anticipation of a cooking competition, I've somewhat become known for makin' bacon and even had the

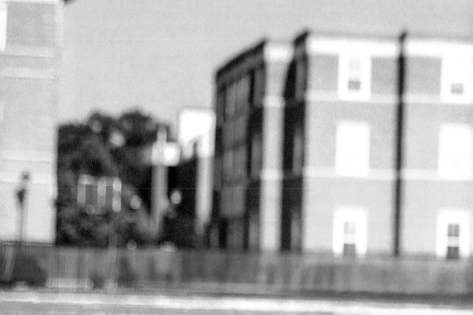

opportunity to share one of my creations live on CBS and NBC morning news programs. Not only is bacon delicious, but you never know when it may lead to some fun, unexpected opportunities :)

Whether you're new to Paleo or an avid follower of the "caveman diet" I think there's something in this book for you, but that's enough jibber-jabbering for the moment. I prefer cooking and photography over writing so why don't I let the food do the talking from here on out? Let's get cookin'!

...on 3
1-2-3 BREAK!!!

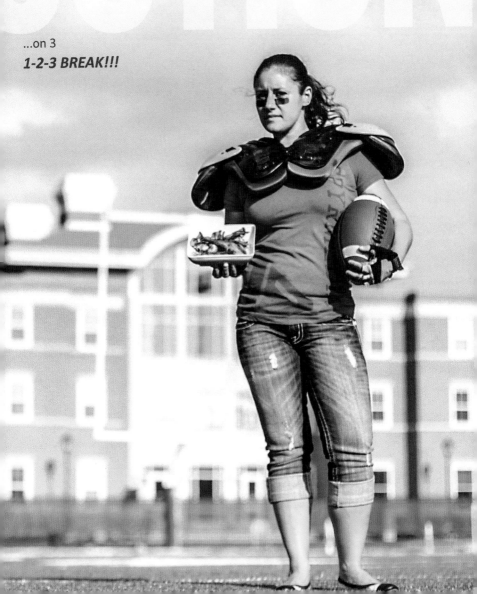

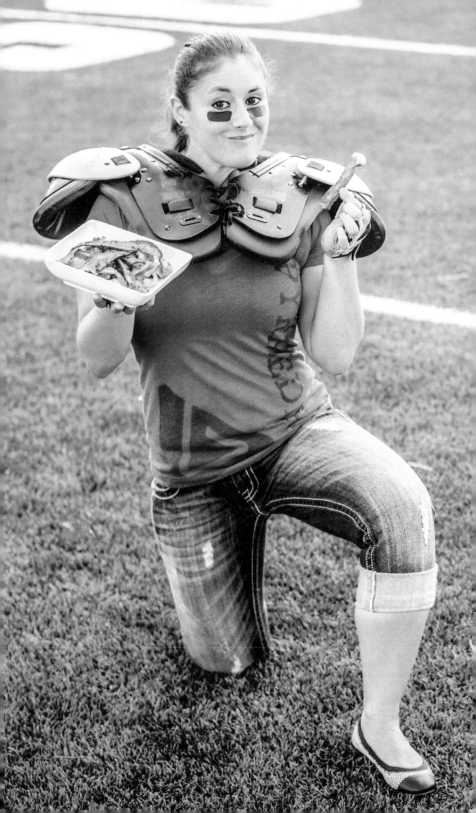

PRE-GAME
APPETIZERS

KICKOFF
SIDEDISHES

GAMETIME
ENTREES

POST-GAME
DESSERTS

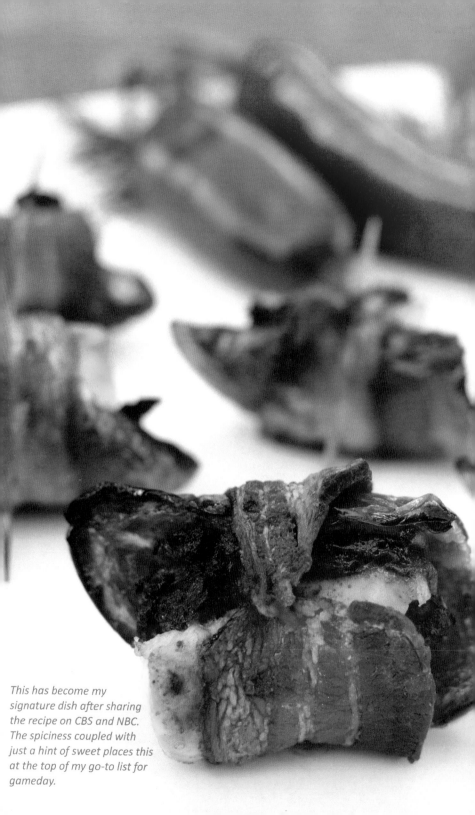

This has become my signature dish after sharing the recipe on CBS and NBC. The spiciness coupled with just a hint of sweet places this at the top of my go-to list for gameday.

BACON WRAPPED CHICKEN CHORIZO POPPERS

SERVES 6

INGREDIENTS:

7.5 ounces beef chorizo
10 jalapeño peppers
5 dates, pit removed and quartered
4-5 chicken tenders, cut into strips the length of the jalapeño peppers
red pepper flakes
10 slices of uncooked sugar-free bacon*
20 toothpicks

DIRECTIONS:

01 Unwrap the chorizo and add it to a frying pan. Cook over medium-high heat until done, making sure to stir throughout. Should be done in 6-8 minutes, 10 minutes max.

02 Cut the tops off the peppers and then slice the pepper in half.

03 Scrape out the seeds from the pepper and discard.
    IMPORTANT: Don't touch your face or eyes while working with the peppers and their seeds. I learned this lesson the hard way. :)

04 If you haven't already, slice each date, remove the pit and cut into quarters.

05 Lay a slice of date on the bottom of each jalapeño pepper.

06 Layer approximately one teaspoon of chorizo over each date.

07 Using kitchen shears, cut a slice of raw chicken tender and lay it across the top of the chorizo. This should not be protruding the top of the pepper. You want little bitty bites so everything has equal flavor.

08 Sprinkle some red pepper flakes across the top of the chicken. Not too much though, unless you want it really spicy.

09 Wrap the stuffed pepper with a half slice of bacon and secure it all in place with a toothpick.

10 Place the bacon wrapped stuffed pepper on a broiler pan and put it in the broiler of the oven.

11 Cook for 8 minutes on each side, flip and cook an additional 6-8 minutes but be sure to keep an eye on them so they don't burn. The second round usually won't take the full 8 minutes.

12 Remove from the oven and transfer to a plate to cool.

Enjoy! :)

* Did you know that not all bacon is created equal? Many packages add sugar as an added ingredient, along with many other unnecessary ingredients. Next time you go to purchase bacon read the ingredient list. It took me a long time to find the perfect bacon and I finally found sugar-free bacon from US Wellness Meats.

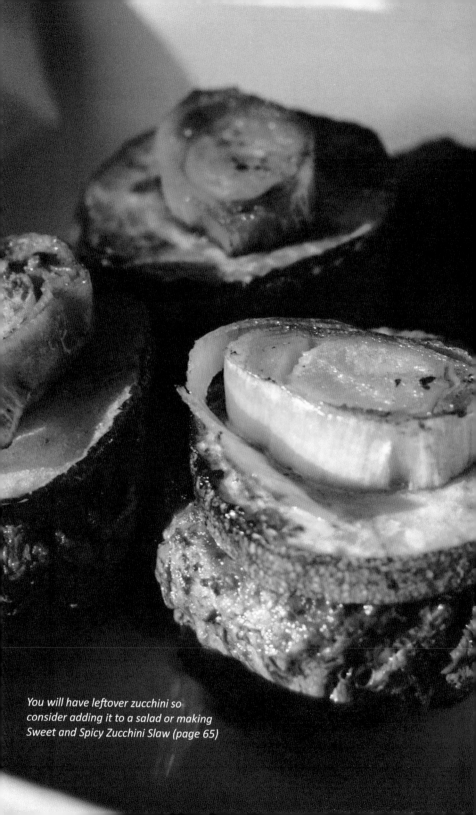

You will have leftover zucchini so consider adding it to a salad or making Sweet and Spicy Zucchini Slaw (page 65)

PRE-GAME
APPETIZER

GRILLED ZUCCHINI-LEEK SLIDERS

INGREDIENTS:

1 lb grass-fed ground beef*
1/4 zucchini, medium to thick slices
1 leek, sliced medium thick

DIRECTIONS:

01 Make small, slider sized beef patties.

02 Add sliders to a grill pan over medium-high heat.

03 While that's cooking slice the zucchini and leek, add to the pan.

04 Flip the sliders and veggies.

05 Transfer to a plate. Top the zucchini on the slider and top the leek on top of the zucchini.

Enjoy! :)

* Grass-fed is always preferred, but if you don't have a stockpile in your fridge or freezer like I do don't let that stop you from enjoying these sliders.

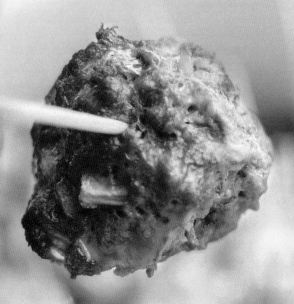

*Burgers are kind of boring so I rarely make
them, but this recipe is short and sweet,
just like me ;)*

ITTY-BITTY BURGER BITES

SERVES 8-10

INGREDIENTS:

1 lb ground beef
1 egg
1/2 red onion, minced
5 garlic cloves, minced
1/2 teaspoon onion powder
1/2 teaspoon garlic powder
1/4 teaspoon tumeric
1/2 teaspoon salt
1/4 teaspoon cumin
1/2 teaspoon chili powder
coconut oil, *optional*
30 toothpicks

DIRECTIONS:

01 Preheat oven to 350° F

02 Add all ingredients to a medium-sized bowl. Using your hands combine and mix well.

03 Use a tablespoon to scoop up a single serving. Using your hands, roll each serving into a ball.

04 Use coconut oil to coat a mini cupcake pan before adding bites or line burger bites up on a parchment paper lined baking tray for easy cleanup.

05 Cook in the oven for 10 minutes. Use the toothpick test to make sure the bites are cooked all the way through. Remove from oven.

06 Once bites are cool, add toothpicks to each ball and serve.

Enjoy! :)

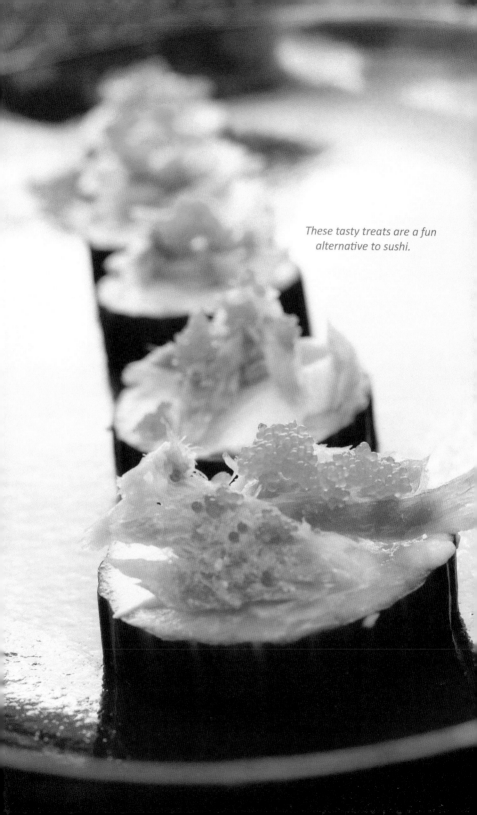

*These tasty treats are a fun
alternative to sushi.*

ROE-TOPPED WHITEFISH CUCUMBERS

SERVES 10-12

INGREDIENTS:

1 english cucumber
1/2 lb smoked whitefish
cream cheese, *optional*
3-4 teaspoons sweetfish roe

DIRECTIONS:

01 Slice cucumber into thin slices.

02 Filet the smoked whitefish, separating the meat from the bones.

03 Smear cream cheese on top of each "cracker" (optional).

04 Top cream cheese with flaked smoked whitefish.

05 Garnish each cracker with a tiny scoop of roe.

Enjoy! :)

ADDITIONAL NOTES:

You can find roe in any Japanese or Korean grocery store. You'll get a large quantity for a very reasonable price.

I prefer to use an English cucumber in this recipe because of its lack of seeds compared to a regular cucumber.

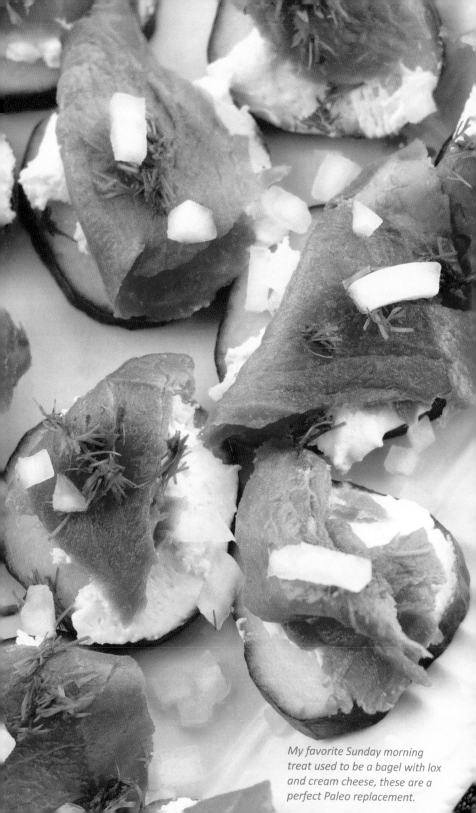

My favorite Sunday morning treat used to be a bagel with lox and cream cheese, these are a perfect Paleo replacement.

NO-BAGEL BITES

SERVES 8-10

INGREDIENTS:

1 english cucumber, sliced
cream cheese, *optional*
wild caught sliced smoked salmon
1-2 plum tomatoes, thinly sliced
1/2 cup onion, minced
fresh dill, chopped *optional*
capers, *optional*

DIRECTIONS:

01 Slice the cucumber into thin slices.

02 Smear cream cheese on top of each cucumber slice, if you choose to use.

03 Layer each cucumber with a half or full slice of salmon (depending on the thickness of the slices).

04 Top each salmon slice with a slice of tomato.

05 Top each tomato with a handful of minced onion.

06 Finish each bagel bite off with a caper or two and a sprinkling of fresh dill.

Enjoy! :)

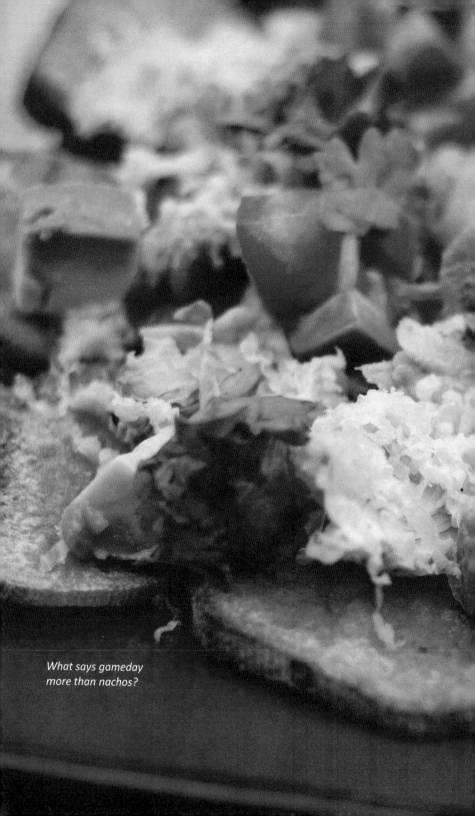

What says gameday more than nachos?

NOT'CHO TYPICAL NACHOS

SERVES 4-6

INGREDIENTS:

2 yuca (cassava root)

2 tablespoons coconut oil

1 lb your choice of meat

1-2 cups shredded cheddar cheese, *optional*

1 green onion, sliced

1 avocado, chopped

1 tomato, chopped

1 cup cilantro, chopped

DIRECTIONS:

01   Preheat oven to 400° F.

02   Remove the exterior of the yuca with a sharp knife. Then slice into 1/8 inch thick chips. Add chips to a large bowl.

03   Melt coconut oil and add to the bowl of yuca chips. Using your hands mix well so chips are coated with coconut oil.

04   Divide yuca chips between two rimmed baking sheets. Elevate the chips by layering them in a single layer across a drying rack on top of the baking sheets.

05   Bake, flipping once, until edges are crisp, 22 to 25 minutes.

06   While the yuca chips are baking fry up some meat. You can use chorizo, bacon, ground beef, ground chicken, ground pork or even shredded chicken or turkey. Use whatever leftover meat you may have. Any protein source is good, cold or warm.

07   Once the yuca chips are done remove from the oven and lay out in a single layer on a platter. Add your choice of hot or cold meat on top of the chips.

08   Shred some cheddar cheese (or your preferred cheese) on top of the meat. (If you shred the cheese while the meat is still hot it will melt nicely when added right away.)

09   Add the remaining ingredients: green onion, avocado, tomato and cilantro along with any other desired toppings for your nachos.

10   Serve immediately.

Enjoy! :)

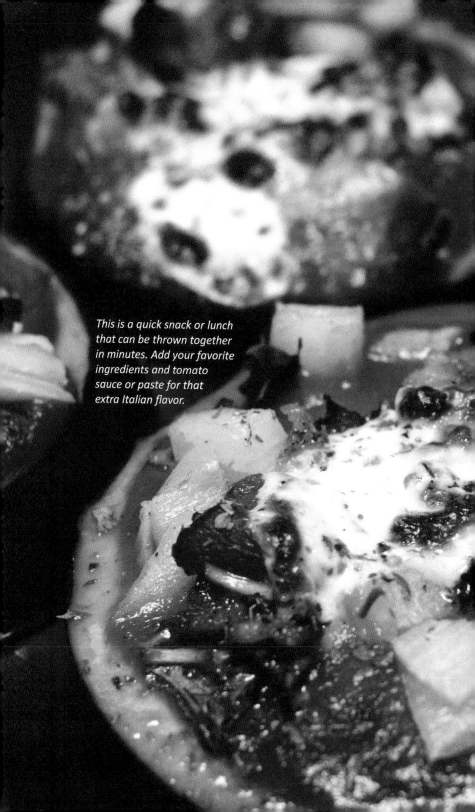

This is a quick snack or lunch that can be thrown together in minutes. Add your favorite ingredients and tomato sauce or paste for that extra Italian flavor.

MINI EGGPLANT PIZZAS

SERVES 4-6

INGREDIENTS:

1 large eggplant, sliced
1/2 cup onion, chopped
2 garlic cloves, minced
1/2 cup fresh basil, shredded
1/2 cup roasted red pepper, chopped
3 slices sugar-free bacon, chopped *optional*

DIRECTIONS:

01 Clean and slice the eggplant so they are 1/4 inch thick.

02 Broil the sliced eggplant for 3 minutes.

03 Remove the eggplant from the oven and flip over.

04 Equally distribute the ingredients between each eggplant slice.

05 Return the eggplant to the broiler for an additional 3-5 minutes.

06 Remove from oven and let cool.

Enjoy! :)

* Did you know that not all bacon is created equal? Many packages add sugar as an added ingredient, along with many other unnecessary ingredients. Next time you go to purchase bacon read the ingredient list. It took me a long time to find the perfect bacon and I finally found sugar-free bacon from US Wellness Meats.

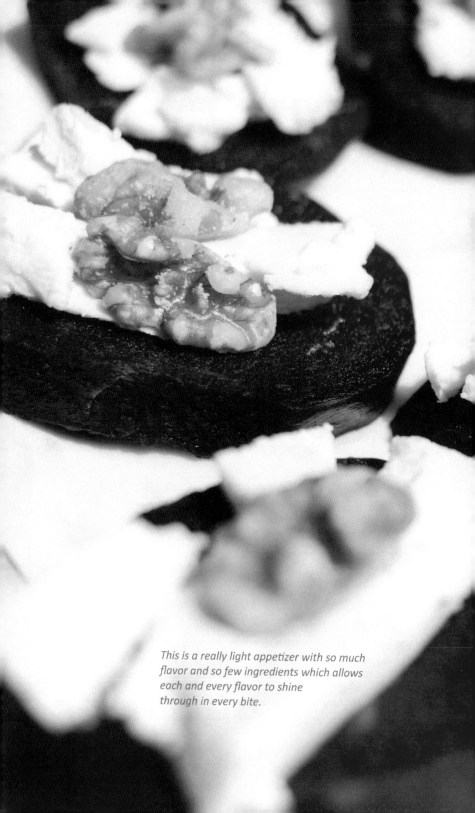

This is a really light appetizer with so much flavor and so few ingredients which allows each and every flavor to shine through in every bite.

PRE-GAME
APPETIZER
BEET BITES

INGREDIENTS:

2 beets, washed and trimmed from stem
1 small log of soft goat cheese
7 raw walnuts, halved

DIRECTIONS:

01　Place beets in a medium size pot and cover with water. Set over high heat until boiling.

02　Boil 25-35 minutes until fork tender.

03　Remove beets from water. When cool enough to handle, slide skin off with your fingers.

04　Slice 1/4 inch thick and arrange on a serving plate.

05　Top each beet slice with a dollop of goat cheese and one walnut half.

Enjoy! :)

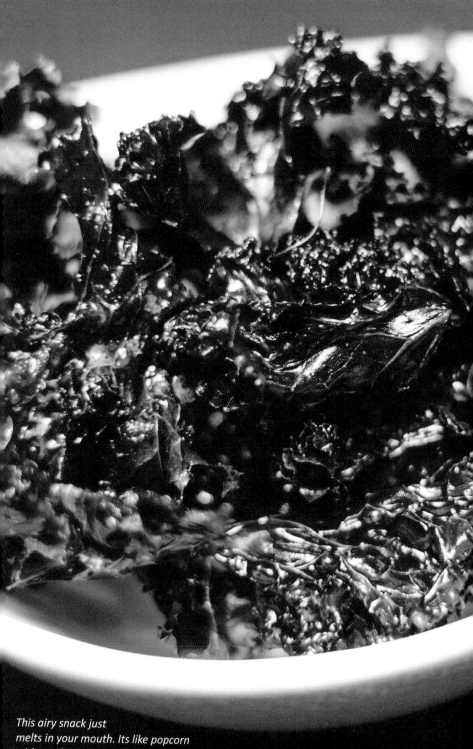

*This airy snack just
melts in your mouth. Its like popcorn
without the grains. Olive oil gives a slightly different flavor than
coconut oil when baked. Feel free to add different seasonings
such as chili powder or garlic power and fancy them up.*

KALE CHIPS

INGREDIENTS:

1 bunch of fresh organic kale
coconut oil
sea salt

DIRECTIONS:

01 Preheat oven to 300° F.

02 Rinse and dry the kale.

03 Tear leaves into medium-to-large pieces. Remove and discard thick stems and center rib.

04 For easy cleanup use 1-2 parchment paper lined rimmed baking sheets. Spread the kale out in a single layer.

05 Lightly drizzle with melted coconut oil and season with sea salt.

06 Bake kale for 15-20 minutes or just until kale chips are crisp, but not browned.

07 Transfer the parchment paper to a wire rack to cool.

Enjoy! :)

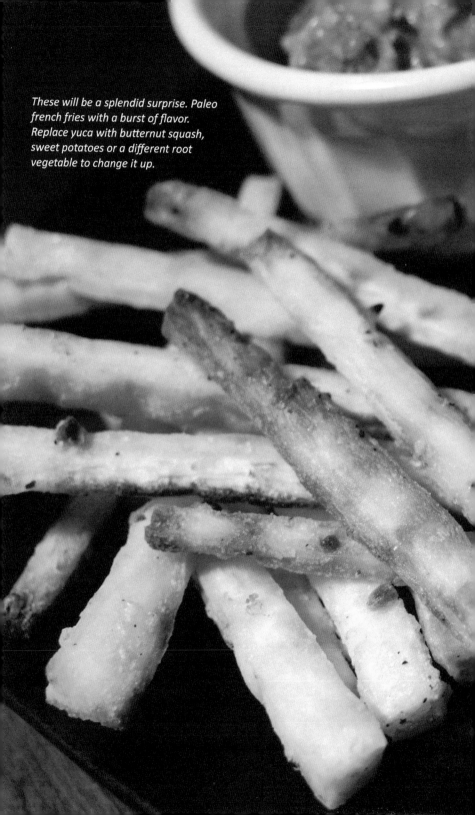

These will be a splendid surprise. Paleo french fries with a burst of flavor. Replace yuca with butternut squash, sweet potatoes or a different root vegetable to change it up.

SEASONED YUCA FRIES

INGREDIENTS:

1 yuca (preferably a long rather than wide yuca root)
2 tablespoons coconut oil, melted
1 tablespoon garlic, minced
1/2 teaspoon onion powder
1 teaspoon salt
1 teaspoon coarse ground black pepper
1/4 cup parmesan cheese, shredded

DIRECTIONS:

01 Preheat oven to 400° F.

02 Cut the ends off the yuca and cut the root into 4 inch chunks. Use a sharp knife to remove the exterior until you see the white flesh. Do this by standing each chunk upright and cutting perpendicular to the ends.

03 Cut each yuca chunk into quarters. Continue to slice each quarter and cut each slice into 1/4-1/2 inch thick fries. Add the fries to a large bowl.

04 Add coconut oil, minced garlic, onion powder, salt, black pepper and shredded parmesan cheese to the bowl.

05 Mix with your hands until everything is evenly distributed.

06 Lay each individual fry on a wire rack on top of a rimmed baking sheet for even baking all around. Organize the fries so they are not touching one another.

07 Bake for 10 minutes then brave the heat of the oven to flip each individual fry over and bake for an additional 10-15 minutes.

08 Remove the fries from the oven and let cool for 5 minutes and serve. (Note: If left for long enough these will become extremely crunchy.)

Enjoy! :)

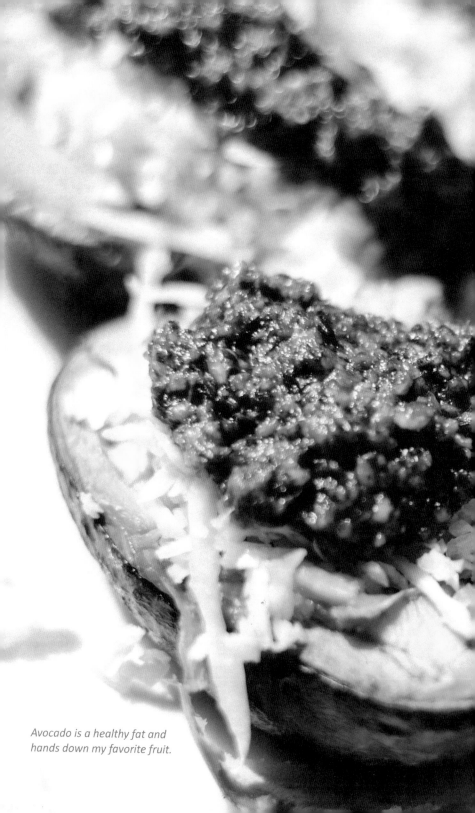

Avocado is a healthy fat and hands down my favorite fruit.

PESTO STUFFED AVOCADO

SERVES 4

INGREDIENTS:

2 avocados
1 cup shredded cabbage
Cashew Pesto (page 53)

DIRECTIONS:

01 Slice avocado in half, remove pit and outer shell. Set aside.

02 Use a food processor to shred cabbage. Stuff each avocado half with shredded cabbage.

03 Top shredded cabbage with a dollop of Cashew Pesto.

Enjoy! :)

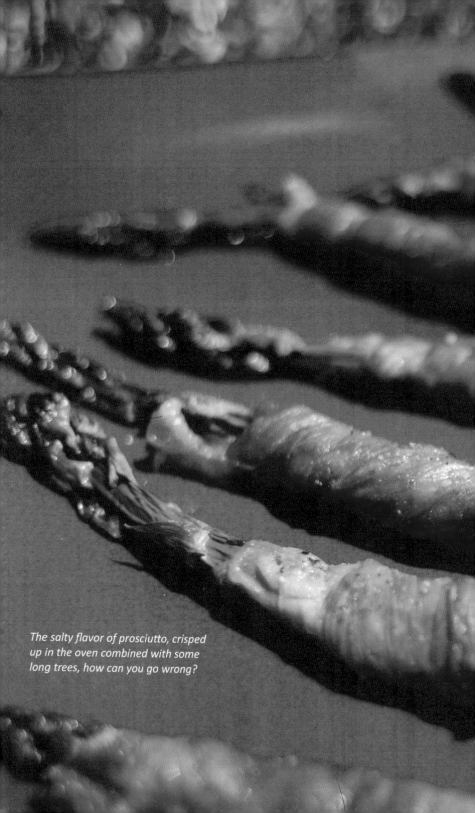

The salty flavor of prosciutto, crisped up in the oven combined with some long trees, how can you go wrong?

PROSCIUTTO WRAPPED ASPARAGUS

SERVES 2-4

INGREDIENTS:

1 **bunch** asparagus
8oz pre-sliced prosciutto
olive oil

DIRECTIONS:

01 Preheat oven to 350° F.

02 Clean and trim asparagus spears.

03 Wrap 1-3 asparagus spears in each slice of prosciutto till you run out of meat.

04 Line a rimmed baking sheet with parchment paper.

05 Lay each asparagus bundle on top of the parchment paper and drizzle olive oil over the top.

06 Bake in the oven for 10 minutes. Check the consistency of the prosciutto, if it's crispy, it's ready, if not leave it in the oven for a couple more minutes.

07 Remove from the oven when ready, let cool.

Enjoy! :)

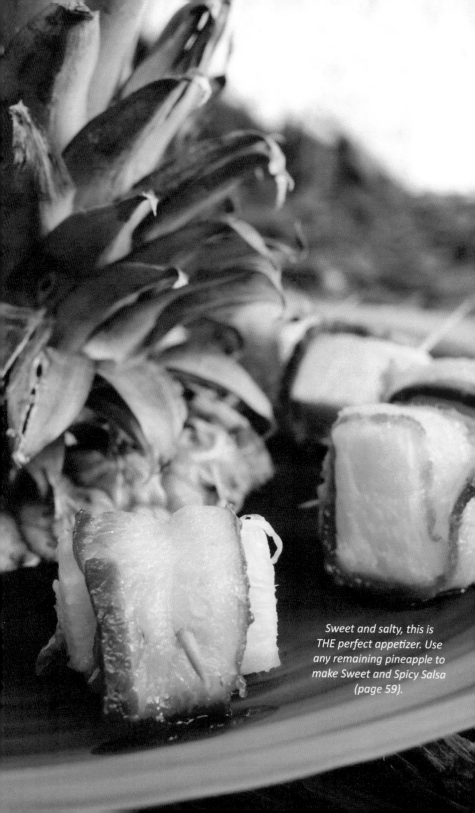

Sweet and salty, this is THE perfect appetizer. Use any remaining pineapple to make Sweet and Spicy Salsa (page 59).

PIGSKIN PINEAPPLE

SERVES 8-10

INGREDIENTS:

15-20 strips of sugar-free bacon
1 pineapple, cubed
coconut oil, melted
toothpicks

DIRECTIONS:

01 Preheat oven to 350° F.

02 Wrap cubed pineapple with half a piece of bacon. Using a toothpick secure it closed.

03 Line a rimmed baking sheet with parchment paper.

04 Lay each wrapped pineapple on top of the parchment paper and drizzle coconut oil over the top.

05 Bake in the oven for 15-20 minutes or until bacon is cooked

06 Remove from the oven when ready, let cool for at least a minute or two before you pop one of those bad boys in your mouth.

07 Serve immediately.

Enjoy! :)

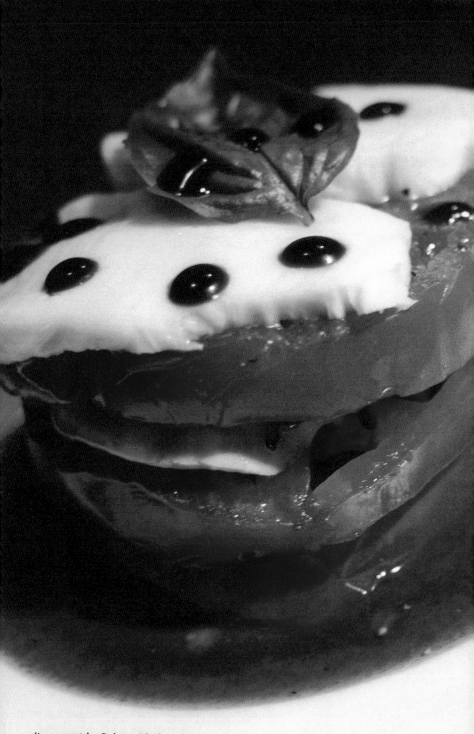

It may not be Paleo with the addition of cheese, but don't let that stop you...I mean unless you're very lactose intolerant ;)

PRE-GAME APPETIZER | CAPRESE TOWER

INGREDIENTS:

4 heirloom (or beefsteak) tomatoes, **sliced 1/2 inch thick**
8 ounces fresh mozzarella cheese, **sliced**
fresh basil leaves
organic balsamic vinegar
salt, **to taste**
pepper, **to taste**
olive oil, **optional**

DIRECTIONS:

01 Starting with a tomato slice, place a mozzarella slice (or two depending on the size) on top of your tomato followed by a full basil leaf. Then drizzle with balsamic vinegar.

02 Continue to stack in this order (tomato, mozzarella, basil) until your desired tower height.

03 Season the last tomato with salt and pepper before topping the final layer with cheese, basil and balsamic vinegar.

04 Drizzle with olive oil, if desired.

Enjoy! :)

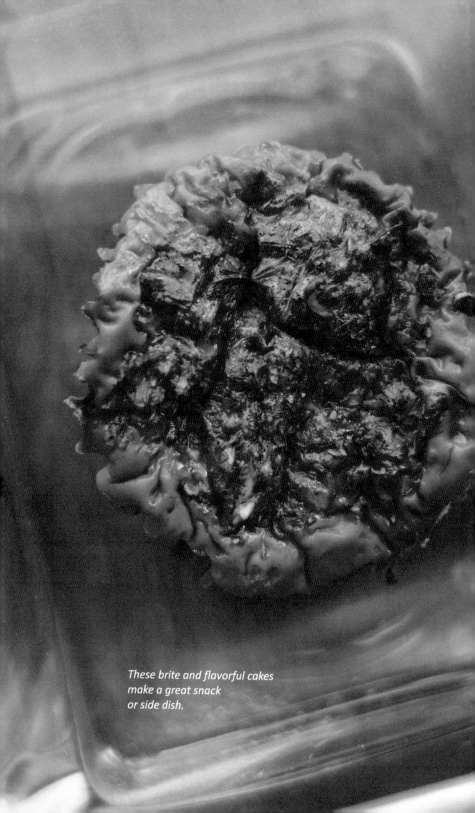

These brite and flavorful cakes make a great snack or side dish.

SPINACH-DILL CAKES

SERVES 8-10

INGREDIENTS:

12 ounces fresh spinach, chopped
1/4 cup fresh dill, chopped
1/2 cup parmesan cheese, finely shredded
2 eggs, beaten
3 garlic cloves, minced
1/4 teaspoon salt
1/4 teaspoon ground black pepper
coconut oil, *optional*

DIRECTIONS:

01 Preheat oven to 400° F.

02 Using a food processor chop fresh spinach in batches until finely chopped.

03 Transfer to a medium size bowl. Add dill, parmesan, eggs, garlic, salt and pepper and stir to combine.

04 Coat a cupcake pan with coconut oil or use parchment baking cups for easy clean up.

05 Divide the spinach mixture among the cups and fill each to the top.

06 Bake the spinach cakes until set, about 20 minutes.

07 Let stand in the pan for 5 minutes to cool.

08 Serve immediately.

Enjoy! :)

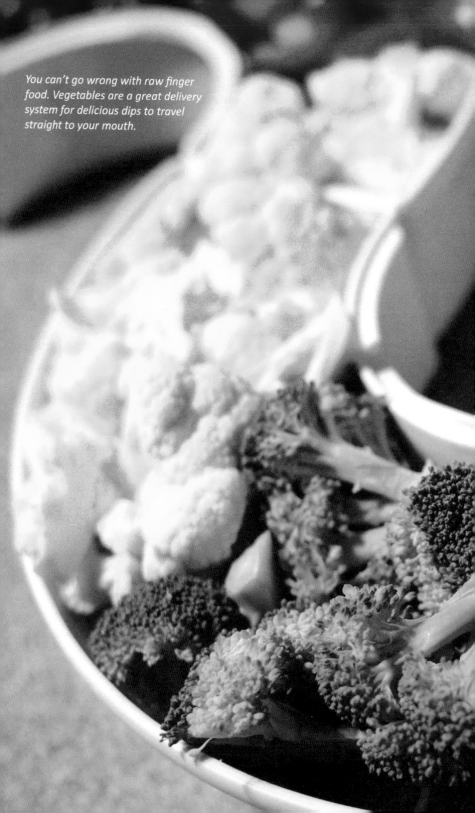

You can't go wrong with raw finger food. Vegetables are a great delivery system for delicious dips to travel straight to your mouth.

PRE-GAME CRUDITÉS
APPETIZER

INGREDIENTS:

4 carrots, sliced
1 head cauliflower florets
1 head broccoli florets
1 zucchini, sliced
6 celery ribs, cleaned and cut into 4 inch sticks
1 pint cherry tomatoes
2 bell peppers, cleaned, trimmed of seeds and cut into strips

ADDITIONAL INGREDIENTS:

1 cucumber, sliced
1 summer squash, sliced
1 fennel bulb, trimmed of frands and cut into strips
1 cup snow peas
1 cup button mushrooms, cleaned
1 cup radishes, cleaned and sliced

DIRECTIONS:

01   Wash, chop and align vegetables on a large serving tray.

02   Serve with Guacamole with a Twist (page 55) & Cashew Pesto (page 53)

Enjoy! :)

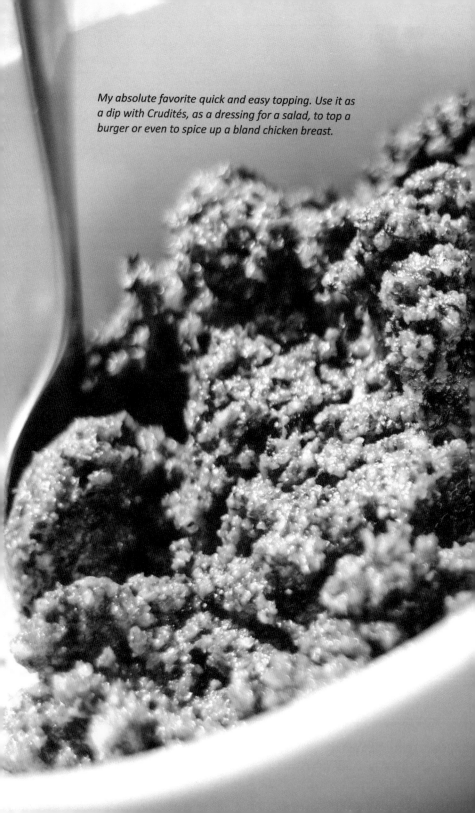

My absolute favorite quick and easy topping. Use it as a dip with Crudités, as a dressing for a salad, to top a burger or even to spice up a bland chicken breast.

CASHEW PESTO

SERVES 6-8

INGREDIENTS:

1 **cup** cashews
4 garlic cloves
1 **cup** basil
olive oil
salt, **to taste**

DIRECTIONS:

01   Add cashews and garlic to a food processor.

02   Add basil to the food processor and blend to mix.

03   While the blade is running add olive oil until it reaches desired consistency.

04   Add salt to taste and blend around 5 seconds to mix together.

Enjoy! :)

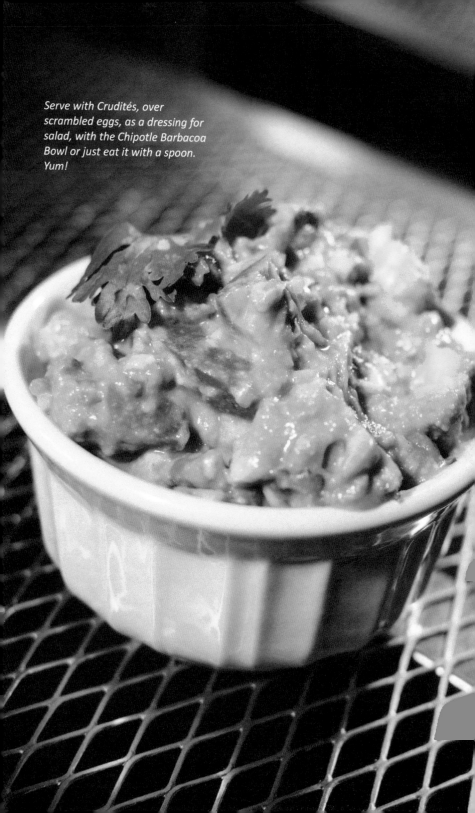

Serve with Crudités, over scrambled eggs, as a dressing for salad, with the Chipotle Barbacoa Bowl or just eat it with a spoon. Yum!

PRE-GAME APPETIZER
GUACAMOLE WITH A TWIST

SERVES 6-8

INGREDIENTS:

3 avocados
1/2 red onion, chopped
5 garlic cloves, minced
1 jalapeño pepper, chopped and seeded
juice of 2 oranges*
1 cup cilantro
sea salt, to taste
2 plum tomatoes, chopped

DIRECTIONS:

01   In a medium bowl add avocado, in large size chunks. Mash with a fork until half smooth and half chunky.

02   Add red onion, garlic, jalapeño pepper, orange juice, cilantro and salt to the bowl. Mix until combined.

03   Add tomatoes prior to serving and mix well until combined.

04   Serve with Crudités (page 51), over scrambled eggs, as a dressing for salad, with the Chipotle Barbacoa Bowl (page 105) or just eat it with a spoon. Yum!

Enjoy! :)

* For a more traditional guacamole, replace the oranges with the juice of 3 limes.

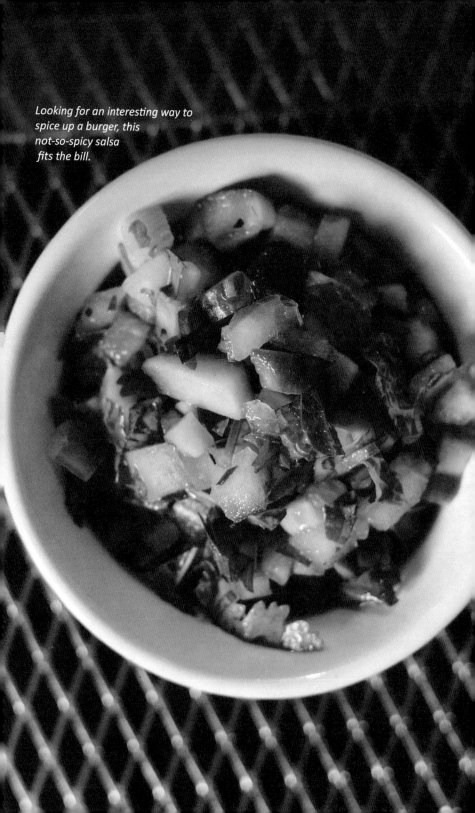

Looking for an interesting way to spice up a burger, this not-so-spicy salsa fits the bill.

CUCUMBER SALSA

SERVES 6-8

INGREDIENTS:

2 persian cucumbers, finely diced
1/2 cup red onion, finely diced
1/4 cup fresh cilantro, chopped
1/4 cup fresh mint, chopped
3 tablespoons fresh lime juice
1 tablespoon olive oil
salt, to taste
pepper, to taste

DIRECTIONS:

01 Mix the cucumber, red onion, cilantro and mint in a medium size bowl.

02 Stir in the lime juice and olive oil.

03 Season with salt and pepper to taste.

04 Add more lime juice if desired.

05 Serve as a topping for bison burgers, grilled chicken, seared tuna or eat it right out of the bowl.

Enjoy! :)

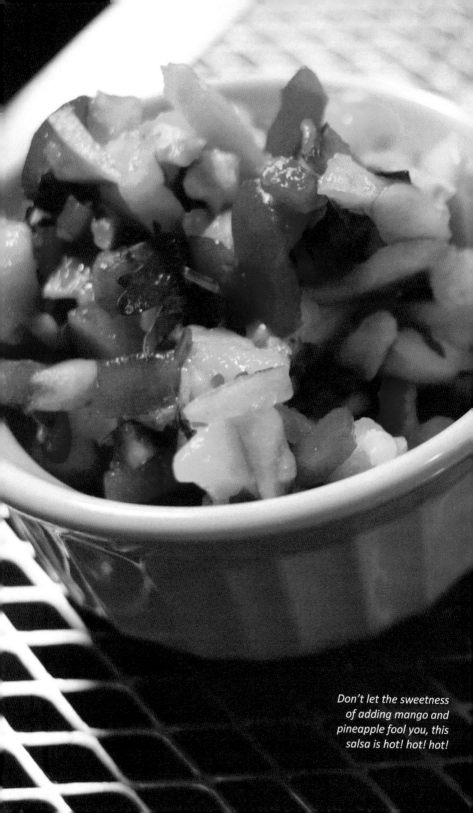

Don't let the sweetness of adding mango and pineapple fool you, this salsa is hot! hot! hot!

SWEET AND SPICY SALSA

SERVES 6-8

INGREDIENTS:

1 cup mango, diced
1 cup pineapple, diced
1/2 cup red pepper, diced
1 whole jalapeño pepper (seeds included), diced
2 tomatillos, chopped
1/4 cup cilantro, chopped
1/3 cup red onion, chopped
1 tablespoon raw honey
juice of 1 lime

DIRECTIONS:

01   Chop everything and add to a medium sized bowl.

02   Serve over grilled fish, chicken or on top of the Chipotle Barbacoa Bowl (page 105).

Enjoy! :)

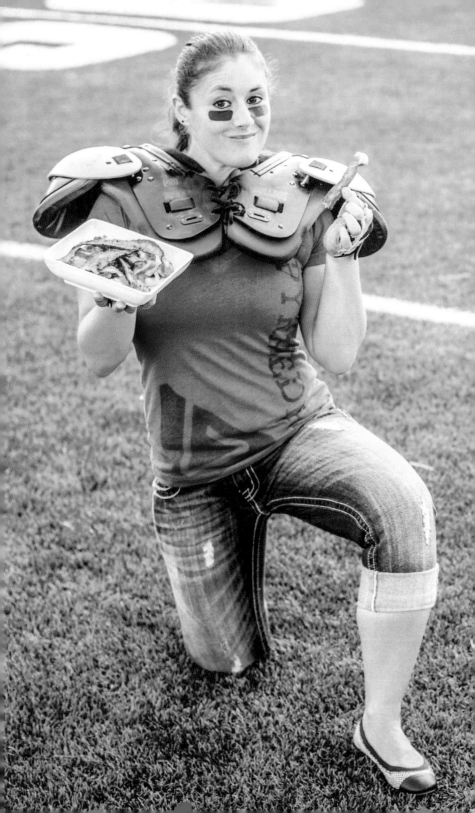

PRE-GAME
APPETIZERS

KICKOFF
SIDEDISHES

GAMETIME
ENTREES

POST-GAME
DESSERTS

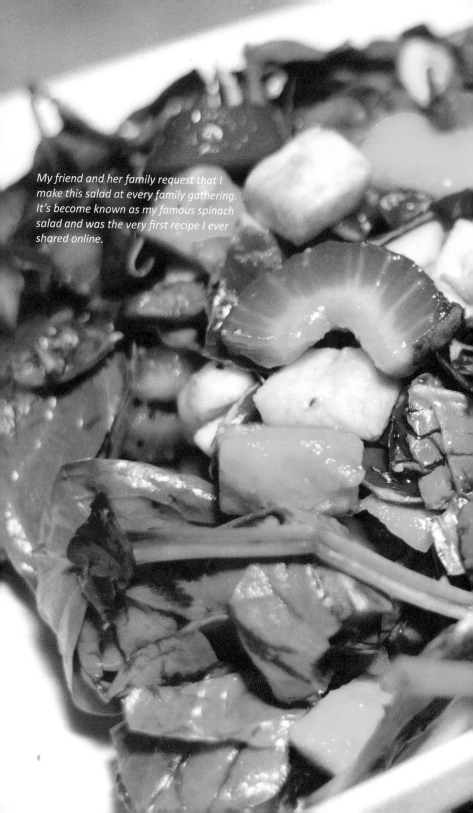

My friend and her family request that I make this salad at every family gathering. It's become known as my famous spinach salad and was the very first recipe I ever shared online.

MARLA'S FAMOUS SPINACH SALAD SERVES 4-6

INGREDIENTS:

1 bunch of fresh organic spinach
1 small head purple cabbage, chopped
16 ounces of fresh strawberries, sliced
1 mango, chopped
8 ounces fresh mozzarella cheese, cubed
1 tablespoon honey
ground black pepper, to taste
balsamic vinegar

DIRECTIONS:

01 Rinse spinach, transfer to a cutting board, chop and transfer to a medium size bowl.

02 Rinse and peal off the outer few layers of cabbage. Transfer to a cutting board and chop the cabbage. Then add it to the top of the spinach in the bowl.

03 Rinse and hull strawberries. Transfer to cutting board and slice. Chop the mango and add both fruits to the bowl.

04 Cube the mozzarella and add to the bowl.

05 Sprinkle ground pepper over the mozzarella, add honey and pour balsamic vinegar from one side to the other across the bowl from front to back.

06 Toss the mixture and taste if more honey or vinegar is necessary.

Enjoy! :)

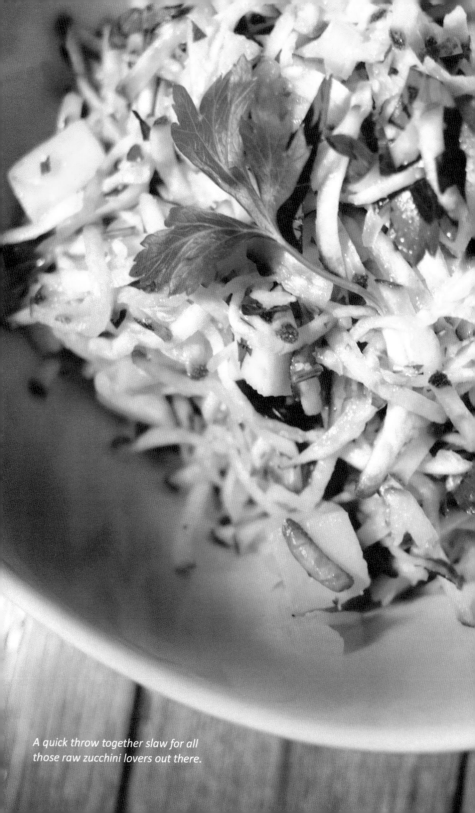

A quick throw together slaw for all those raw zucchini lovers out there.

SWEET AND SPICY ZUCCHINI SLAW

SERVES 4-6

INGREDIENTS:

1 1/2 cups shredded zucchini
2 banana peppers, chopped
1 mango, chopped
1/2 cup flat leaf parsley, chopped
1/4 cup olive oil
garlic salt, to taste
oregano, to taste

DIRECTIONS:

01   Use a food processor to shred the zucchini. Add to a medium size strainer and let sit while you add the remaining ingredients to a medium sized mixing bowl.

02   Rinse and chop the banana peppers. If you want more spicy of a slaw keep the seeds, if not remove them.

03   Slice the mango and chop into medium size chunks.

04   Add the zucchini to the mango & peppers.

05   Finely chop the parsley and add it to the top of the mix.

06   Sprinkle the olive oil, garlic salt and oregano on top.

07   Mix it all together and serve.

Enjoy! :)

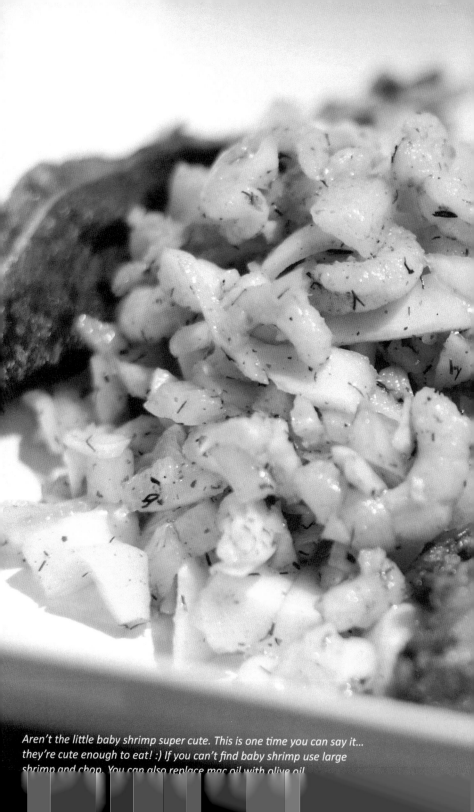

Aren't the little baby shrimp super cute. This is one time you can say it... they're cute enough to eat! :) If you can't find baby shrimp use large shrimp and chop. You can also replace mac oil with olive oil.

BABY SHRIMP COLESLAW

SERVES 2-3

INGREDIENTS:

1/2 cabbage, chopped
1 onion, chopped
4 garlic cloves, chopped
2 cups cooked wild organic pink baby shrimp
1 tablespoon dried dill
1 tablespoon dried oregano
1 teaspoon celery salt
1 teaspoon jerk pork seasoning
2/3 cup macadamia nut oil

DIRECTIONS:

01 Combine all ingredients in a large mixing bowl.

02 Mix to combine, add more macadamia nut oil if desired.

Enjoy! :)

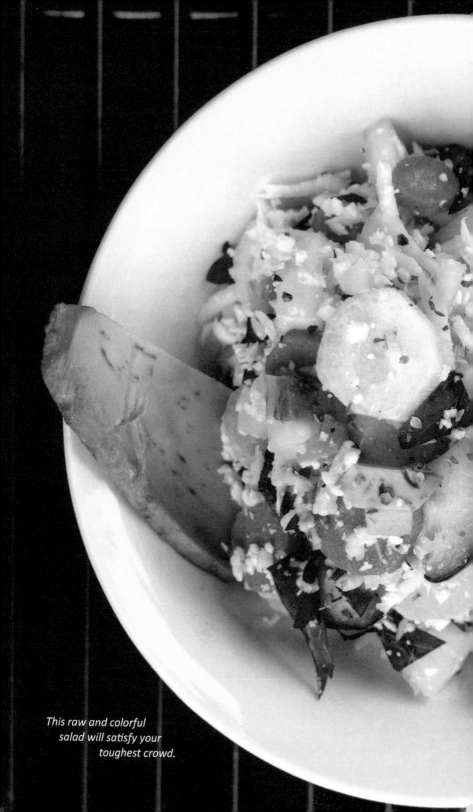

This raw and colorful
salad will satisfy your
toughest crowd.

CAULIFLOWER RAINBOW SALAD

SERVES 10–12

INGREDIENTS:

1/2 head cauliflower, shredded
6 rainbow carrots, sliced*
2 radish, chopped
1 cup flat leaf parsley, chopped
1/2 yellow pepper, chopped
1 english cucumber, chopped
1 pint grape tomatoes
1 onion, chopped
1 teaspoon oregano
juice of 1 lime
2 tablespoons olive oil
1 avocado, chopped

DIRECTIONS:

01   Shred cauliflower in a food processor and add to a large size bowl.

02   Add remaining ingredients to the bowl.

03   Right before serving chop the avocado and add to the bowl, mix well and serve.

Enjoy! :)

* Rainbow carrots come in all different colors; purple, yellow, white, orange, etc. If you can't find them regular carrots will work just fine. :)

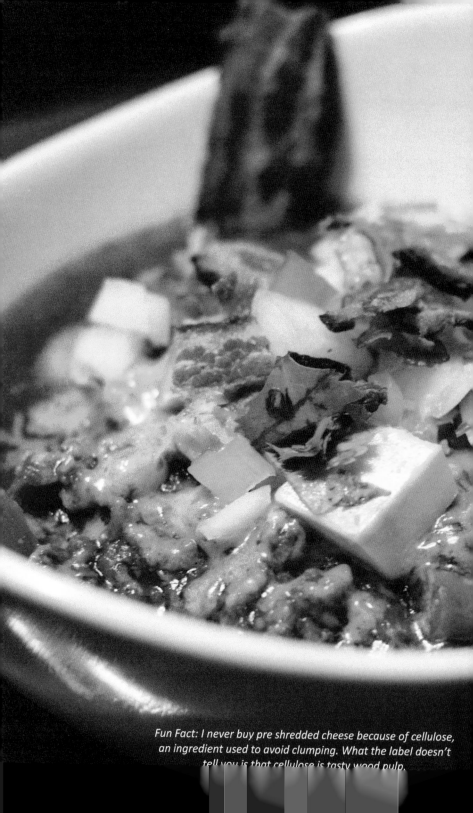

Fun Fact: I never buy pre shredded cheese because of cellulose, an ingredient used to avoid clumping. What the label doesn't tell you is that cellulose is tasty wood pulp.

PRIME TIME CHILI

SERVES 8-10

INGREDIENTS:

1 onion, chopped
5 garlic cloves, sliced
1 large carrot, sliced
3 organic celery ribs, chopped
10 strips of sugar-free bacon, divided*
1 green pepper, chopped
1 serrano pepper, sliced
4 thai chili peppers, ends chopped off and sliced
2 pounds grass-fed ground beef or bison
26 ounces chopped tomatoes**
26 ounces strained tomatoes**
2 tablespoons chili powder
1/8 teaspoon paprika
1/8 teaspoon oregano
1/8 teaspoon cumin
1 avocado, chopped
1/4 cup cilantro, chopped
2 green onions, sliced
shredded cheddar cheese, *optional***

DIRECTIONS:

01 Let's start with a little prep work. Chop the onion, garlic, carrot and celery but keep about a 1/4 cup of onion off to the side to use for topping.

02 Using kitchen sheers cut 6 strips of bacon into about 2 inch pieces.

03 Using a large pot over medium heat add the bacon. (I used a 5qt pot) Give it a swirl with a wooden spoon and once the pieces start to get more solid and some bacon fat has coated the pan add the onion, garlic, carrot and celery pieces. Mix everything around a bit.

04 While that's working on it's own chop the remaining veggies (green pepper, serrano pepper and thai chili peppers) and as you finish chopping each one, add them to the pot. Mix everything around with the wooden spoon until combined well.

05 After a couple minutes move everything in the pot over to one side and throw in the meat. Mix it around in that half of the pot until the meat is mostly browned. Then combine everything together so you have a good mixture of meat and veggies.

06   Add the chopped tomatoes and strained tomatoes, chili powder, paprika, oregano and cumin and give it one final swirl with the spoon, mix until combined well.

07   Bring the mixture to a boil.

08   Reduce the heat to medium-low and let the chili simmer for 30-60 minutes (or longer). If you're looking for a quick dish 30 minutes is plenty of time for the meal to be ready to eat. The longer you let it simmer, the spicier the chili will get but don't let it simmer too long or you may need to add some water.

09   While the chili is doing it's thing, fry up the last 4 strips of bacon to use for a topping, and feel free to pop one of those bad boys in your mouth while you're waiting. (Although then you may want to have more than 4 strips prepared.)

10   Serve topped with some shredded cheddar, fresh avocado, chopped onion, green onion, a little cilantro and some bits of bacon.

Enjoy! :)

* Did you know that not all bacon is created equal? Many packages add sugar as an added ingredient, along with many other unnecessary ingredients. Next time you go to purchase bacon read the ingredient list. It took me a long time to find the perfect bacon and I finally found sugar-free bacon from US Wellness Meats.

** I use Pomi brand strained and chopped tomatoes. It's BPA free and the ingredients are what they're supposed to be, tomatoes, nothing more & nothing less.

*** To avoid cellulose I use a block of Kerrygold White Cheddar and shred it myself.

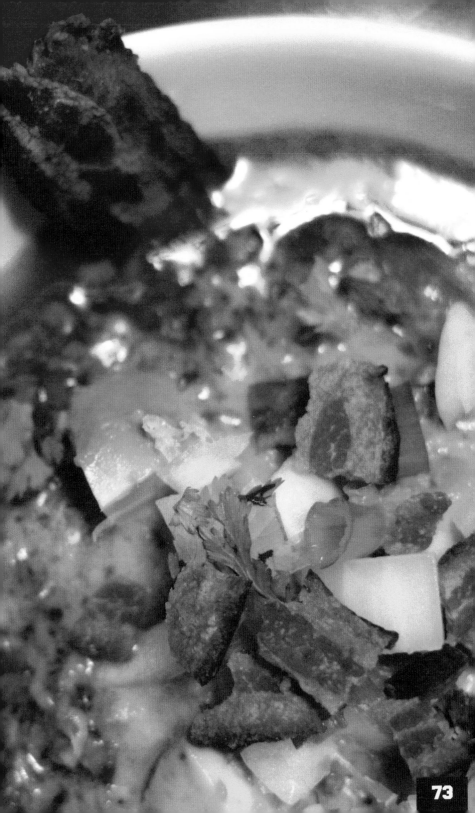

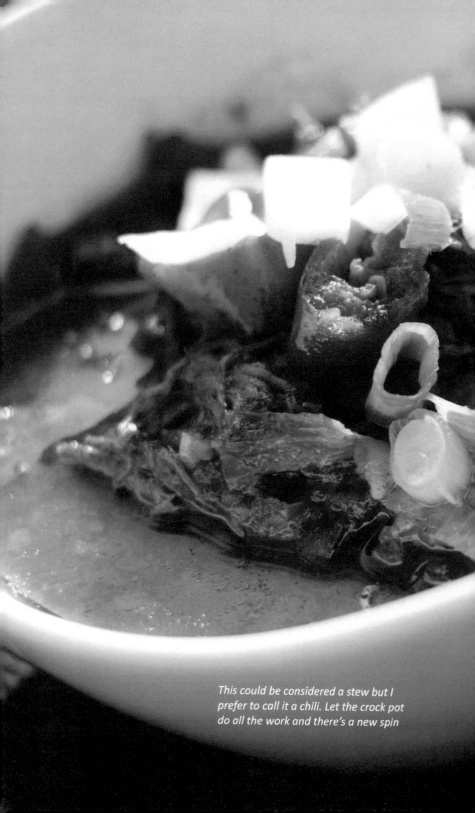

This could be considered a stew but I prefer to call it a chili. Let the crock pot do all the work and there's a new spin

MEAT & POTATOES CHILI

SERVES 8-10

INGREDIENTS:

3.5 **pound** chuck roast
1 **cup** button mushrooms, **sliced**
1 head of garlic
1 sweet potato,
3 **tablespoons** chili powder
3 jalapeño peppers, **sliced**
26 **ounces** chopped tomatoes*
1 **tablespoon** cumin
1 **tablespoon** coriander
1 **tablespoon** oregano
1 **cup** water

DIRECTIONS:

01   In a large frying pan brown the chuck roast, cooking for around 4-5 minutes on each side.

02   Transfer roast to crockpot. Add all remaining ingredients on top of roast.

03   Cook on high for 6 hours.

Enjoy! :)

* I use Pomi brand chopped tomatoes. It's BPA free and the ingredients are what they're supposed to be, tomatoes, nothing more & nothing less.

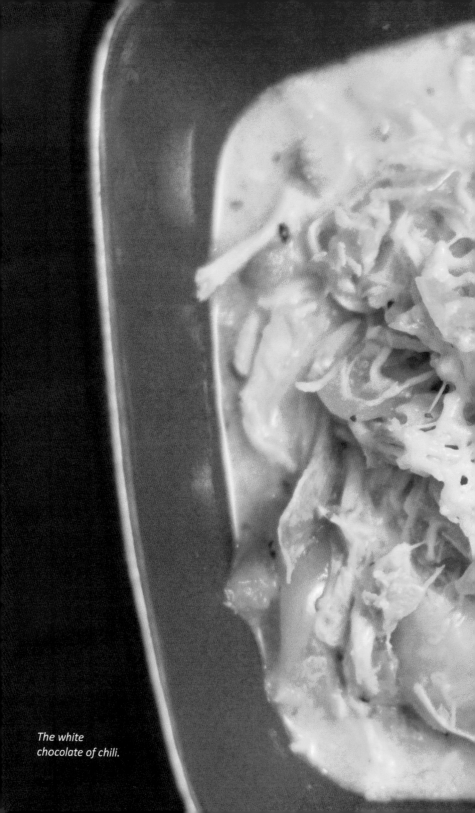

The white chocolate of chili.

WHITE CHILI

SERVES 6-8

INGREDIENTS:

2 lbs chicken breast
1 white onion, chopped
4 celery ribs, chopped
8-10 garlic cloves, sliced
1 can unsweetened coconut milk
1 cup organic chicken broth
1 yellow pepper, chopped
3 parsnips, sliced
onion powder
garlic powder
oregano
cumin
shredded asiago cheese, *optional*

DIRECTIONS:

01 In a large frying pan brown the chicken breast on each side.

02 Transfer chicken to the crockpot. Add all remaining ingredients on top, minus the cheese.

03 Cook on high for 6 hours.

04 Using two forks shred the chicken breast.

05 Serve with shredded asiago cheese on top.

Enjoy! :)

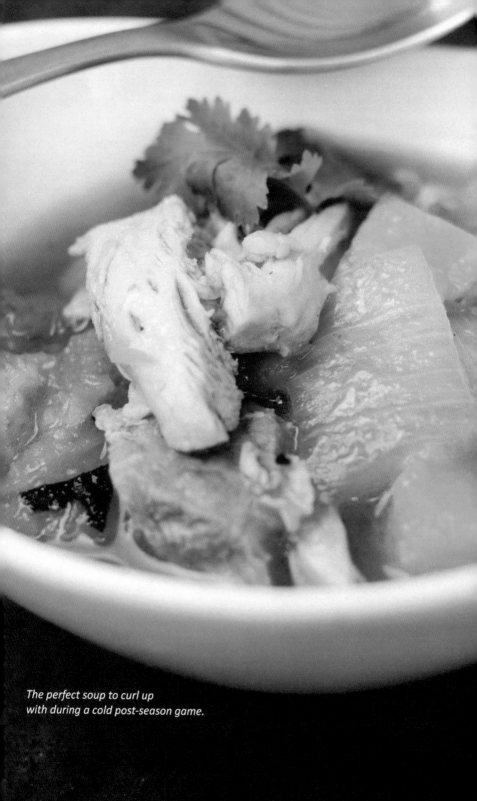

The perfect soup to curl up with during a cold post-season game.

KICKOFF SIDEDISHES
ROASTED CHICKEN & BUTTERNUT SOUP

SERVES 4-6

INGREDIENTS:

4 bone-in chicken thighs
1 medium butternut squash, peeled, seeded and diced
1 onion, diced
2 tablespoons olive oil
salt, to taste
pepper, to taste
4 cups organic chicken broth
1/4 teaspoon cumin
1/4 teaspoon coriander
juice of 1 lemon
fresh cilantro

DIRECTIONS:

01 Preheat the oven to 425° F.

02 Arrange in a single layer the chicken, squash and onion across 1-2 rimmed baking sheets. Drizzle with olive oil and season with salt and pepper.

03 Roast until squash and chicken are cooked through, about 30 minutes.

04 Transfer chicken to a plate and let cool

05 Transfer squash and onions to a medium pot and combine with chicken broth, cumin and coriander.

06 Bring to a simmer over medium-high heat.

07 While waiting for soup to simmer cut the meat into small pieces.

08 With a potato masher, mash some vegetables until soup is thick and chunky.

09 Add the chicken to the soup.

10 Stir in lemon juice.

11 Serve topped with fresh cilantro.

Enjoy! :)

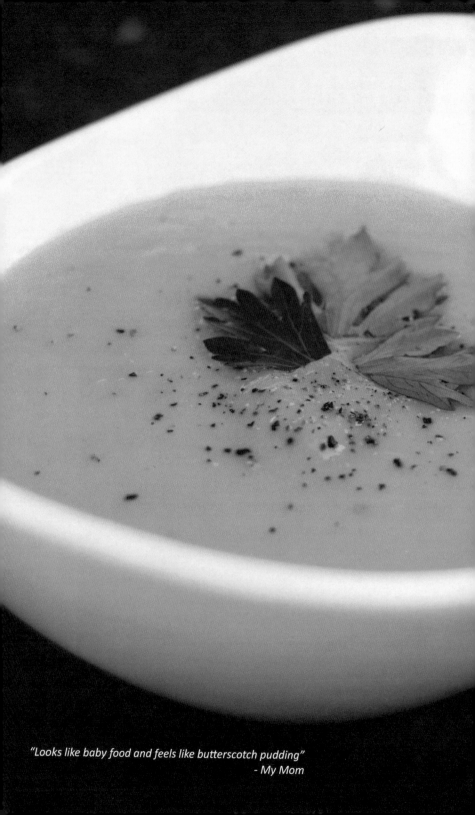

"Looks like baby food and feels like butterscotch pudding"
- My Mom

CREAMY CARROT SOUP

SERVES 8-10

INGREDIENTS:

3 tablespoons butter, divided
1 onion, chopped
1 1/2 lbs sweet potatoes, peeled and chopped
3 1/2 cups water
3 cups organic chicken broth
1 lb carrots, chopped (approximately 3-4 regular size carrots)
1/2 teaspoon salt
1/4 teaspoon ground black pepper
2 tablespoons flat-leaf parsley, chopped

DIRECTIONS:

01 Melt 1 tablespoon of butter in a large pot over medium heat.

02 Add onion and cook for 4 minutes or until tender, stirring occasionally.

03 Move onion to the side of the pan and add the remaining 2 tablespoons of butter in the open space in the pan.

04 Increase heat to medium high and cook for 1 minute or until butter begins to brown.

05 Add sweet potatoes, water, broth and carrot, bring to a boil.

06 Cover, reduce heat to medium-low and simmer for 35 minutes or until vegetables are tender.

07 Add the soup mixture, in stages, to a blender. Remove center piece of blender, to allow steam to escape. Secure lid and place a clean towel over opening in the blender to avoid splatter. Blend until smooth. Pour soup into a large bowl.

08 Repeat procedure with remaining soup mixture until done.

09 Stir in salt and pepper.

10 Serve topped with fresh parsley.

Enjoy! :)

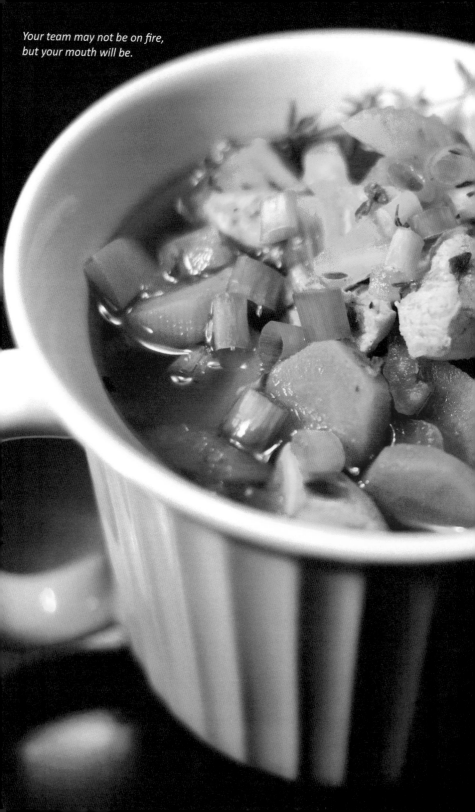

Your team may not be on fire,
but your mouth will be.

CAYENNE KICKS YOUR ASS CHICKEN SOUP

SERVES 3-4

INGREDIENTS:

1-2 tablespoons butter
3 carrots, chopped
salt, to taste
ground black pepper, to taste
ground red pepper (cayenne pepper)
3 celery ribs, chopped
1/2 onion, chopped
1/2 orange pepper, chopped
1/2 yellow pepper, chopped
1 quart organic chicken broth
2 cups water
5 garlic cloves, chopped
1.5 lbs chicken tenders, cubed
1/2 cup fresh thyme
1/2 cup green onions, sliced

DIRECTIONS:

01 Add butter to a large pot and melt over medium heat.

02 Chop carrots and add them to the pot.

03 Add a few shakes of salt, pepper and cayenne to the carrots. Stir a bit and let it sit while you chop the celery, onion and peppers. Be sure to return to the pot every few minutes to continue to stir.

04 Add the onions and celery to the pot, mix to combine.

05 Using kitchen sheers cut the chicken tenders into cubes and add to a bowl.

06 Add the orange & yellow peppers to the pot, mix to combine. Let the mixture combine for a few minutes before moving on to the next step.

07 Add the chicken broth and water to the mixed vegetables.

08 Chop the garlic and add to the bowl with the chicken. Sprinkle some salt and pepper and a generous amount of cayenne pepper into the bowl. Use your hands to mix everything together.

09 Add the chicken mixture to the pot, stir to combine.

10 Add the chopped fresh thyme and mix everything together. Turn up the heat to medium high, cover and bring to a boil. Simmer for 15-20 minutes.

11 Chop the green onion and set aside.

12 Pour the soup into a bowl, top with sliced green onion and enjoy! :)

Enjoy! :)

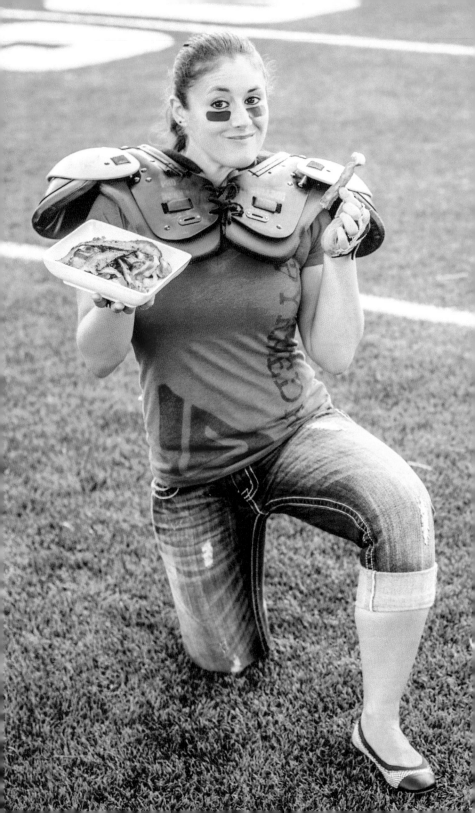

PRE-GAME
APPETIZERS

KICKOFF
SIDEDISHES

GAMETIME
ENTREES

POST-GAME
DESSERTS

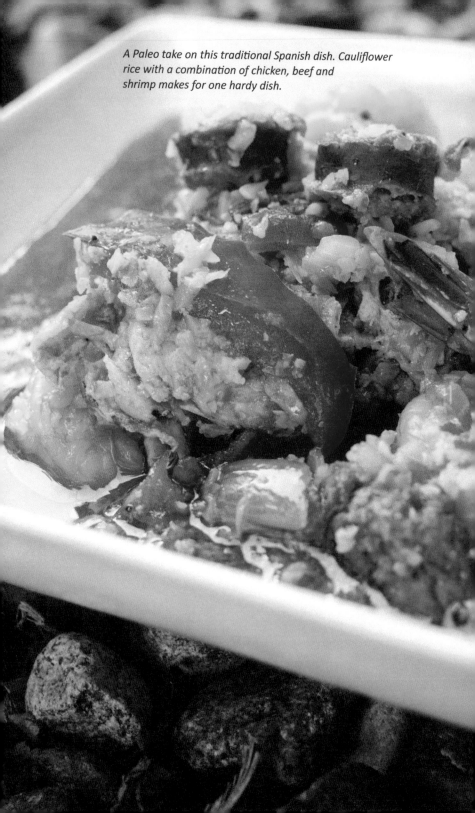

A Paleo take on this traditional Spanish dish. Cauliflower rice with a combination of chicken, beef and shrimp makes for one hardy dish.

GAME DAY PAELLA

SERVES 4-6

INGREDIENTS:

choice of fat: butter, ghee, coconut oil, etc.
4 chicken thighs and 2-4 chicken breast
salt, to taste
ground black pepper, to taste
1 lb your choice of meat (beef chorizo, grass-fed ground beef or bison)
1 red bell pepper, ribs and seeds removed, thinly sliced
1/2 small onion, chopped
3 garlic cloves, minced
14.5 ounces diced tomatoes
32 ounces organic chicken broth
1 head of cauliflower, shredded
1/2 lb peeled and de-veined jumbo shrimp (thaw if frozen)

DIRECTIONS:

01   Season chicken with salt and pepper.

02   In a heavy-bottomed pot, heat your choice of fat over medium-high heat.

03   Working in batches, cook chicken (be sure not to overlap the chicken in the pot) until browned, 7 to 8 minutes, turning once.

04   Transfer the chicken to a plate and set aside. In the same pan cook the ground meat over medium high heat. Be sure to break it up and stir occasionally.

05   Add the bell pepper, onion, garlic and tomatoes (with their juice) to the pot; season with salt and pepper. Cook, stirring occasionally, until liquid has pretty much evaporated, 5-7 minutes.

06   Add broth, chicken and shredded cauliflower rice; bring to a boil.

07   Reduce to a simmer; cover and cook 8-10 minutes.

08   Add shrimp, submerging them in liquid. Cover and cook until shrimp are opaque throughout, 4 to 6 minutes.

Enjoy! :)

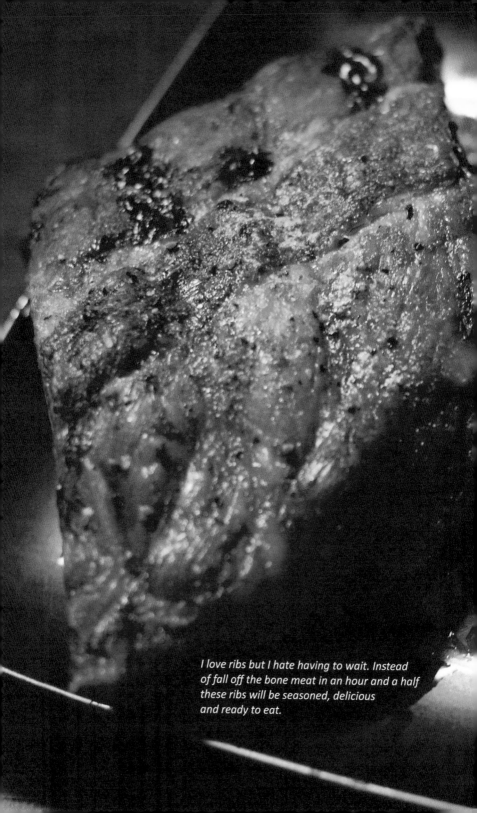

I love ribs but I hate having to wait. Instead of fall off the bone meat in an hour and a half these ribs will be seasoned, delicious and ready to eat.

THE IMPATIENT MAN'S SEASONED RIBS

SERVES 3-4

INGREDIENTS:

2 racks of ribs
salt, to taste
pepper, to taste
garlic powder
grass-fed butter

DIRECTIONS:

01 Preheat the oven to 350° F.

02 Cut the ribs into manageable pieces (3-4 ribs per cluster).

03 Sprinkle salt, pepper and garlic powder (in that order) on the bone side first, then flip over and sprinkle ingredients on the opposite site, leaving the ribs bone side dow n on a thin baking sheet.

04 Roast ribs for 30 minutes in the oven. (Switch baking sheets in the oven, if using multiple sheets. If not using multiple baking sheets, rotate the sheet.)

05 Roast ribs for another 30 minutes.

06 After the first hour is complete, slice chunks of butter on each set of ribs and lay on top of the ribs while in the oven.

07 Roast ribs for final 30 minutes.

08 Take ribs out of the oven and let cool for 20-25 minutes.

Enjoy! :)

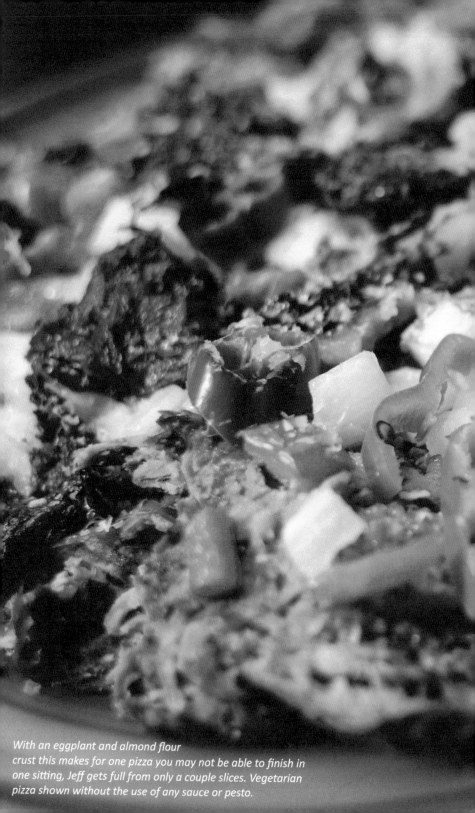

With an eggplant and almond flour
crust this makes for one pizza you may not be able to finish in
one sitting, Jeff gets full from only a couple slices. Vegetarian
pizza shown without the use of any sauce or pesto.

GAMETIME ENTREES

PRIMAL PIZZA

INGREDIENTS:

1/2 cup almond flour or almond meal
1/4 cup parmesan cheese
3 garlic cloves, minced
1 egg white
1 medium to large size eggplant (approximately 1 lb grated)
salt, to taste
ground black pepper, to taste
oregano, to taste
butter
1 onion, chopped
3-5 garlic cloves, minced
1 jalapeño pepper, sliced
1 portobello mushroom, sliced
1 green pepper or red pepper, sliced
oregano
tomato sauce, tomato paste, pizza sauce or pesto *optional*
mozzarella cheese, *optional*
mild ground italian sausage, ground beef, bacon, *optional*

DIRECTIONS:

01 Preheat the oven to 450° F.

02 Use a food processor to grate the eggplant.

03 Add the grated eggplant to the bottom of a medium size mixing bowl.

04 Measure out the almond meal and cheese and add the cloves of garlic to the bowl along with the egg white.

05 You can add any other extra ingredients or seasonings to the crust. I usually add salt, pepper and oregano to taste.

06 Combine all the ingredients, mix well.

07 Roll parchment paper out over a pizza stone, or large cookie tray, to bake your crust on.

08 Butter the parchment paper everywhere the crust will be. (You'll see why this is important when you get to step 12.)

09 Pour the pizza dough mixture out on the parchment paper. Using your hands, flatten out the dough into your desired shape, whether that's a square, rectangle or circle it doesn't matter.

10 Put in the oven for 15 minutes.

11 While the crust is cooking, pan fry the italian sausage (or whatever meat may need to be cooked) and cut up all the veggies you'd like to use for your toppings.

12 Pull the crust out of the oven and use the parchment paper to help you flip the crust over. Discard the parchment paper. At this point the crust should be slightly cooked through. Not much of the crust should stick to the paper since you buttered it.

13 Put the crust back in the oven for another 5 minutes, still at 450° F. (After 5 minutes, if the crust edges don't look completely done, give it a minute or two more, but keep your eye on it so it doesn't burn.)

14 Pull the crust out of the oven and let it cook for 10 minutes. This will increase how firm the dough gets, prior to adding the toppings.

15 Add the topping ingredients of your choice. If using some type of tomato sauce or pesto I usually start with that and finish with any lightweight ingredients such as fresh basil and seasonings.

16 Put the pizza back in the oven for another 10 minutes, now at 350° F. If you added cheese, once it's melted you know it's done.

17 Take the pizza out of the oven and let it cool for 5 minutes, then cut and eat.

Enjoy! :)

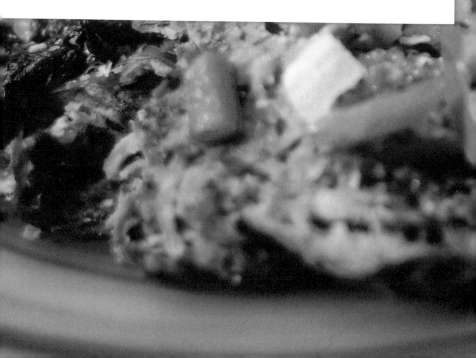

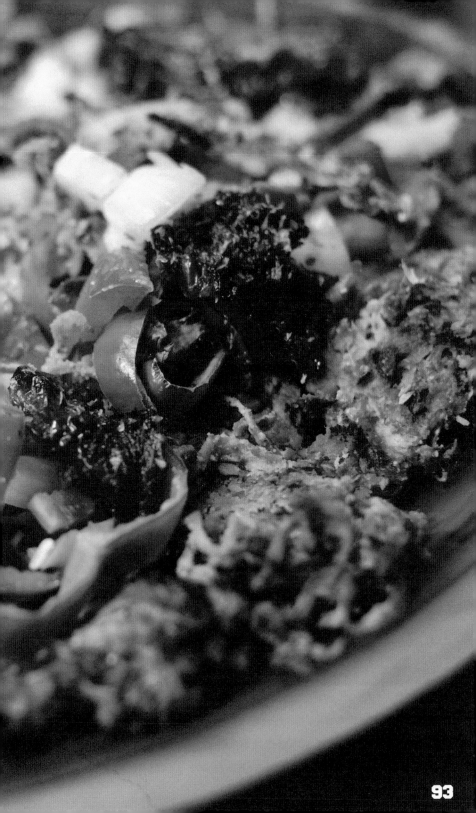

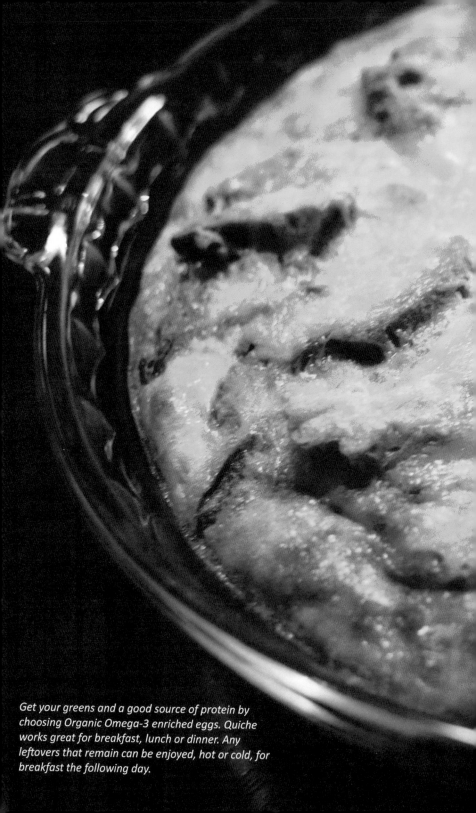

Get your greens and a good source of protein by choosing Organic Omega-3 enriched eggs. Quiche works great for breakfast, lunch or dinner. Any leftovers that remain can be enjoyed, hot or cold, for breakfast the following day.

GO-GREEN CRUSTLESS QUICHE

SERVES 3-4

INGREDIENTS:

grass-fed butter
1 onion, chopped
2 jalapeño peppers, sliced
1 bunch of asparagus
1/4 cup sharp cheddar cheese, *optional*
6 eggs
salt, to taste
ground black pepper, to taste
1 avocado, sliced

DIRECTIONS:

01 Preheat your oven to 350° F.

02 Set a medium size frying pan to medium heat and melt the butter, then add the chopped onions.

03 While the onion is cooking chop the jalapeño peppers and add to the pan.

04 While the onion and peppers are cooking, be sure to stir every so often, rinse off the asparagus and chop into 1 inch pieces.

05 If you see the onion starting to brown, turn the heat to low.

06 Crack the eggs into a large size mixing bowl and whisk.

07 Add the fresh asparagus to the eggs. Then add the pepper and onion, straight from the pan, into the large mixing bowl. Sprinkle with salt and pepper to taste.

08 Shred the cheese directly into the bowl, eyeball about 1/4 of a cup.

09 Mix it all together and pour into your favorite baking dish. (I prefer my 10-inch fluted round pie dish.)

10 Then slice one avocado into thin slices and layer across the top.

11 Shred a shallow layer of finely graded cheese across the top of the avocado. This will provide a nice golden top once it melts.

12 Bake in the oven for 25 minutes.

13 Make sure all the sides have browned a bit along the edges and use the toothpick test to make sure the center has completely set.

Enjoy! :)

Note: So many combinations can be made with quiche, throw in some garlic or really any veggies you'd like. Remember that some vegetables will cause the quiche to produce more liquid, depending on what you add.

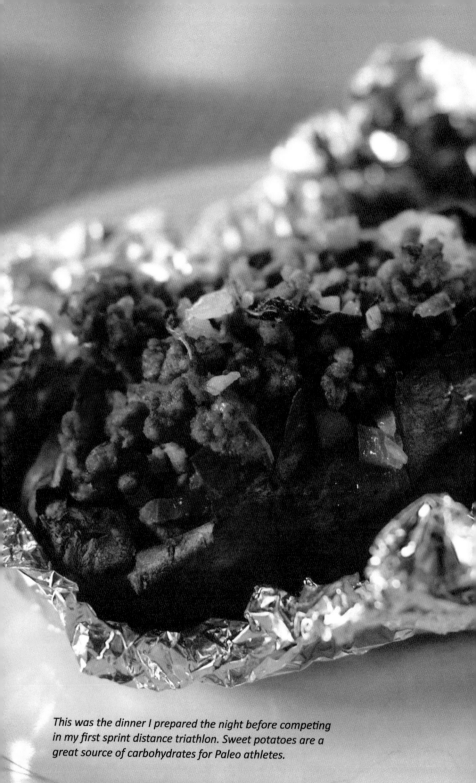

This was the dinner I prepared the night before competing in my first sprint distance triathlon. Sweet potatoes are a great source of carbohydrates for Paleo athletes.

STUFFED SWEET POTATOES SERVES 4+

INGREDIENTS:

4 **large** sweet potatoes
1 **tablespoon** grass-fed butter
1 onion, **chopped**
1 fennel bulb, **core removed and chopped**
4 garlic cloves, **diced**
2-3 **teaspoons** fresh thyme
salt, **to taste**
ground black pepper, **to taste**
1 **lb** ground pork

DIRECTIONS:

01 Preheat the oven to 350° F.

02 Wash and stab the sweet potatoes with a fork a few times, wrap in aluminum foil and bake for at least 1 hour.

03 In a large frying pan, heat butter and sauté onion and fennel for approximately 1 minute.

04 Add garlic and half of the herbs.

05 Sauté for several minutes to blend flavors.

06 Salt and pepper to taste. Remove and transfer to a plate.

07 In the same pan, add pork and brown until cooked, stirring frequently.

08 Return onion mixture to the pan with the browned meat and continue to cook for 5 minutes.

09 Add remaining fresh thyme. (Add small amount of water if necessary to keep the mixture moist.)

10 Adjust seasoning to taste.

11 Once the potatoes are done, carefully slice each one open and scoop some of the pork mixture inside. If potatoes were pre-cooked, heat the stuffed potatoes in the oven together at 350° F until warm. If cooking everything at once remove potatoes from oven, let cool for 5-10 minutes. Then stuff and eat.

Enjoy! :)

Note: This recipe can be made using ground beef, ground turkey, ground pork, or even left off and replaced with more vegetables to make it vegetarian/vegan friendly.

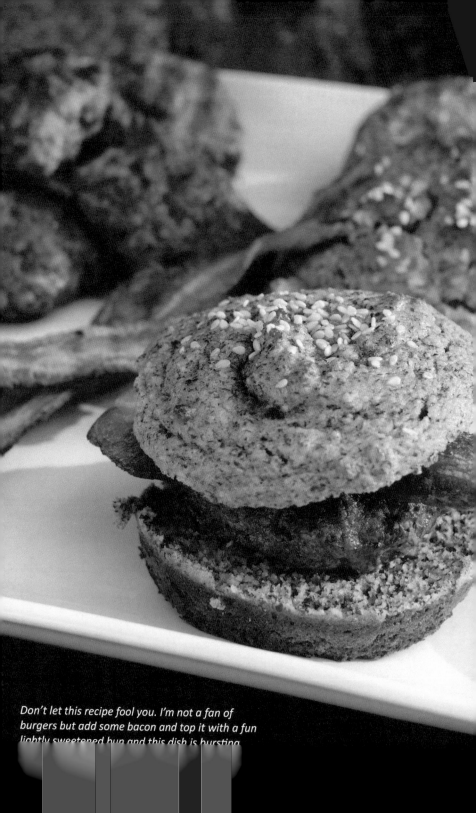

Don't let this recipe fool you. I'm not a fan of burgers but add some bacon and top it with a fun lightly sweetened bun and this dish is bursting

BACON BURGERS WITH ALMOND MEAL BUNS

SERVES 4

INGREDIENTS (BURGERS):

1 lb grass-fed ground beef
salt, to taste
ground black pepper, to taste
8-10 slices of bacon, because you know 2 will go straight in your mouth ;)

INGREDIENTS (BUNS):

1 1/2 cup almond flour
2 eggs
1 teaspoon raw honey
1/2 teaspoon baking soda
1/2 teaspoon salt
8 teaspoons of water
sesame seeds, for garnish

DIRECTIONS:

01 Preheat the oven to 350° F.

02 In a bowl mix almond flour, eggs yolks, baking soda, salt and honey.

03 Beat the egg whites until stiff peaks form.

04 Add almond flour mixture to the egg whites and using a hand mixer add water to combine.

05 Pour batter into a muffin top pan and garnish with sesame seeds.

06 Bake 10 minutes or until golden brown. Remove from oven and let cool.

07 Use your hands to form 4 patties with the ground beef. (Using 1 pound of meat you can make between 4-6 burgers however the bun recipe only produces 4 buns so load on the meat!)

08 Salt and pepper both sides of the burgers before adding them to a frying pan. Cook over medium heat between 3-5 minutes per side, depending on how rare or well done you'd like them.

09 Transfer burgers to a plate and cook strips of bacon in same pan.

10 Slice open the buns, and create your burger with two slices of bacon each.

Enjoy! :)

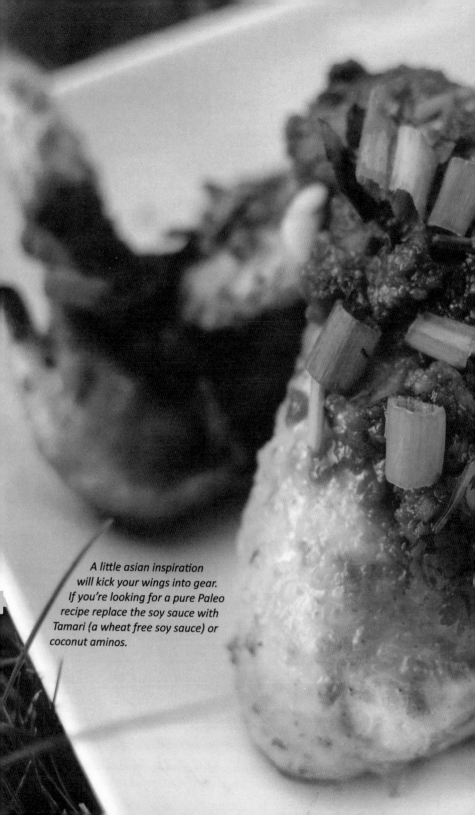

A little asian inspiration will kick your wings into gear. If you're looking for a pure Paleo recipe replace the soy sauce with Tamari (a wheat free soy sauce) or coconut aminos.

STICKY THAI CHICKEN WINGS

SERVES 2

INGREDIENTS (WINGS):

1 1/2 lbs chicken wings
2-3 tablespoons coconut oil

INGREDIENTS (SAUCE):

1/4 cup rice vinegar
3 tablespoons chili paste
1/2 cup canned unsweetened coconut milk
5 garlic cloves, minced
juice of 1 lime
1 heaping tablespoon almond butter
1/2 tablespoon soy sauce

INGREDIENTS (GARNISH):

1/4 cup fresh cilantro, chopped
1 green onion, chopped

DIRECTIONS:

01 Preheat the oven to 325° F.

02 Pat chicken wings completely dry then season with salt and pepper.

03 Combine remaining ingredients for sauce in a medium sized bowl and mix.

04 Heat a large oven-safe skillet over medium high heat with coconut oil.

05 Add chicken wings and sear for 2-4 minutes per side. Remove wings and set on a plate, then reduce heat to medium.

06 Add chili sauce mixture and bring to a boil. Let simmer for 1-2 minutes before adding wings back into the sauce.

07 Place skillet in the oven and bake for 25-30 minutes.

08 Remove and spoon the sauce over the top of the wings, then garnish with cilantro and green onion.

Enjoy! :)

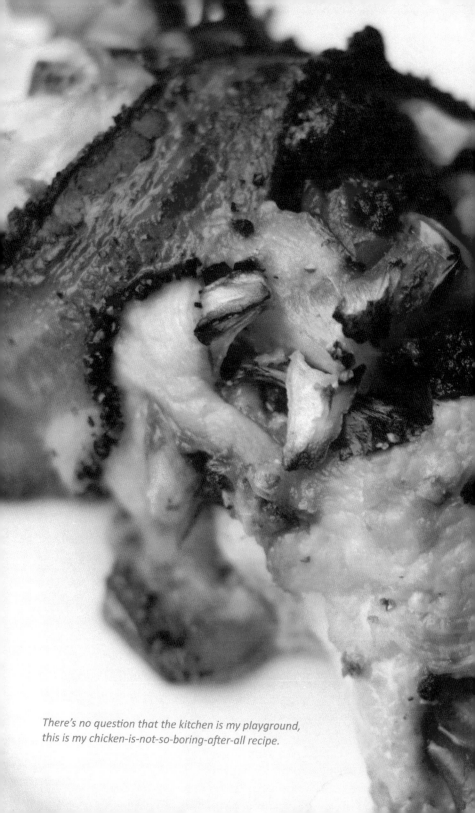

*There's no question that the kitchen is my playground,
this is my chicken-is-not-so-boring-after-all recipe.*

BACON ROCK-N-ROLL CHICKEN

SERVES 4

INGREDIENTS:

4 large chicken breast
salt, to taste
ground black pepper, to taste
oregano, to taste
1 cup spinach, chopped
1/4 cup orange pepper, chopped
1/4 cup red pepper, chopped
1/4 cup onion, chopped
3 garlic cloves, minced
4-8 slices of sugar-free bacon
4-8 toothpicks

DIRECTIONS:

01 Preheat the oven to 350° F.

02 Lay individual chicken breast between wax or parchment paper. Using the flat end of a meat tenderizer, pound chicken until very thin.

03 Season chicken breast with salt, pepper and oregano.

04 Add a handful of spinach, orange pepper, red pepper, onion and garlic to the top of the seasoned chicken.

05 Roll the chicken breast closed.

06 Wrap the stuffed chicken breast with 1-2 slices of bacon. Secure closed with 1-2 toothpicks.

07 Repeat steps 1-5 above for the remaining chicken breast.

08 Add the bacon-wrapped stuffed chicken to a large oven proof baking dish.

09 Bake for 30-40 minutes or until chicken and bacon are done.

10 Remove from oven and let cool 10-15 minutes.

Enjoy! :)

* Did you know that not all bacon is created equal? Many packages add sugar as an added ingredient, along with many other unnecessary ingredients. Next time you go to purchase bacon read the ingredient list. It took me a long time to find the perfect bacon and I finally found sugar-free bacon from US Wellness Meats.

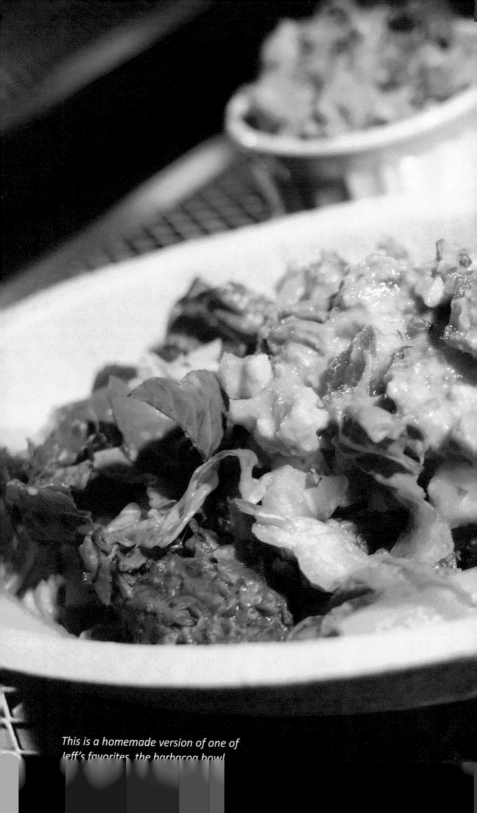

This is a homemade version of one of Jeff's favorites, the barbacoa bowl.

CHIPOTLE BARBACOA BOWL

SERVES 3-4

INGREDIENTS:

2-2 1/2 pound chuck roast
5 chipotle chiles in adobo sauce
1/4 cup red wine vinegar
juice of 1 lime
8 garlic cloves, minced
1 teaspoon cumin
1 teaspoon oregano
1 teaspoon course ground black pepper
1 teaspoon sea salt
1/2 cup organic chicken broth
1 bay leaf
1 head of romaine lettuce, shredded
1 yellow pepper, thinly sliced
1 onion, thinly sliced
Sweet and Spicy Salsa (page 59)
Guacamole With a Twist (page 55)

DIRECTIONS:

01   In a large frying pan over medium high heat sear all sides of the roast until browned.

02   While the meat is browning, add the chipotle chiles, vinegar, lime juice, garlic, cumin, oregano, salt and black pepper to a food processor and blend until smooth.

03   Place the meat into a crockpot and pour the adobo sauce from the food processor over the meat.

04   Pour in the chicken broth and add a bay leaf.

05   Cook on high heat for 6 hours.

06   Shred the meat using two forks and turn the heat to warm.

07   Serve in a bowl over shredded romaine lettuce, with sliced pepper and onion. Top it off with some Sweet and Spicy Salsa and Not Your Typical Guacamole to tame the flame from the salsa. ;)

Enjoy! :)

Fun Fact: A chipotle chile is a jalapeño pepper that has been dried and smoked and usually canned in a spicy sauce called adobo.

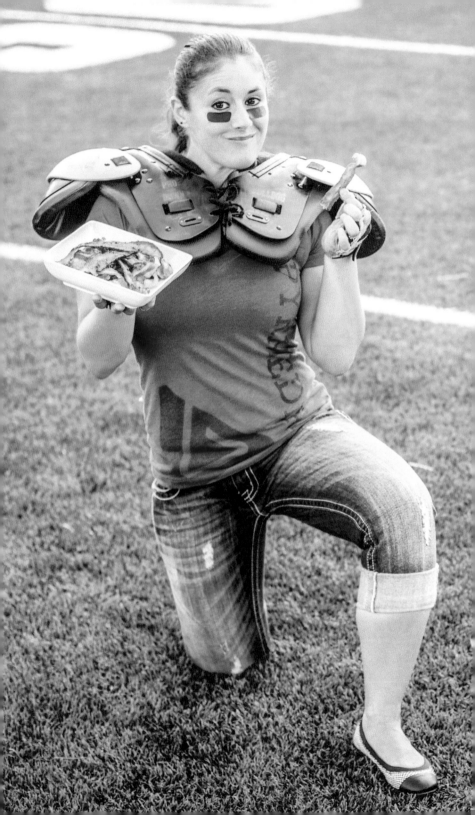

PRE-GAME
APPETIZERS

KICKOFF
SIDEDISHES

GAMETIME
ENTREES

POST-GAME
DESSERTS

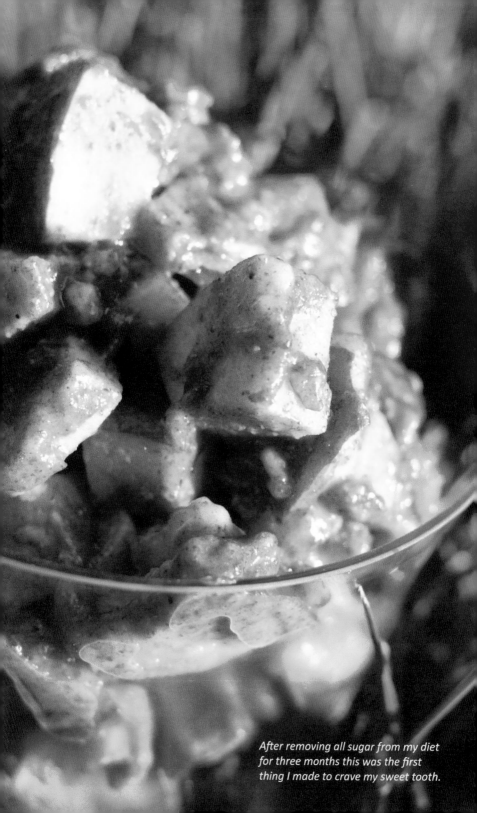

After removing all sugar from my diet for three months this was the first thing I made to crave my sweet tooth.

APPLE PIE IN A BOWL

SERVES 2

INGREDIENTS:

1 banana
1 fuji apple
2 tablespoons of chunky almond butter
1 tablespoon cinnamon
1/4 teaspoon nutmeg

DIRECTIONS:

01 Slice the banana and add it to a medium sized bowl.

02 Slice the apple, then chop it into medium size squares (comparable in size to the distance from your knuckle to the tip of your thumb) and add it to the bowl with the banana.

03 Add the almond butter, cinnamon and nutmeg to the mixture.

04 With a large spoon, probably the one you used to scoop the almond butter, mix everything together. Taste to see if more almond butter or cinnamon is needed.

05 Then take that bowl and spoon and walk anywhere you want and enjoy your apple pie in a bowl.

Enjoy! :)

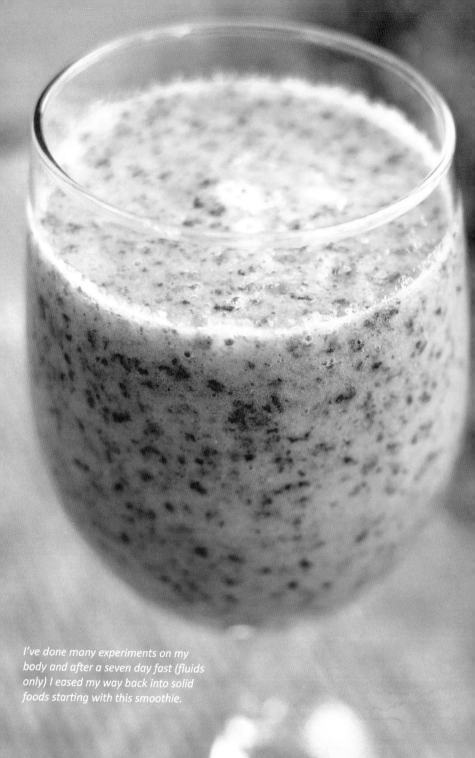

I've done many experiments on my body and after a seven day fast (fluids only) I eased my way back into solid foods starting with this smoothie.

BANANA-PEAR GREEN SMOOTHIE

SERVES 2

INGREDIENTS:

2 bananas
2 **ripe** organic pears
1-2 cups organic baby spinach
1 persian cucumber
1/2 cup of egg whites
4-5 ice cubes

DIRECTIONS:

01   Peal and add the bananas to the bottom of the blender.

02   Slice the pear into 3-4 large pieces, cutting away from the core and seeds in the center.

03   Wash and chop off the ends of the cucumber and add in 2-3 chunks to the blender.

04   Wash and add spinach to the top.

05   Add ice and blend until smooth.

06   Blend everything to the consistency of your choice. We like our smoothies with a little bit of texture, meaning I don't like them to be so smooth that they become a juice.

07   Pour and serve.

Enjoy! :)

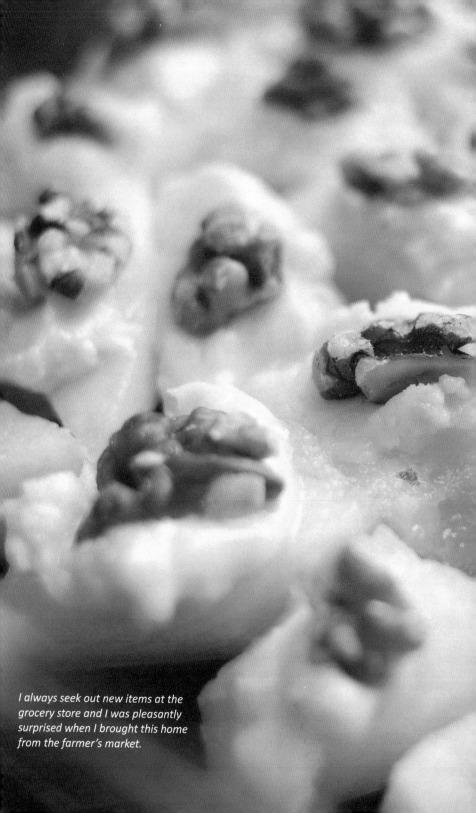

I always seek out new items at the grocery store and I was pleasantly surprised when I brought this home from the farmer's market.

SANTA CLAUS COCONUT BITES

SERVES 10-12

INGREDIENTS:

1/2 santa claus melon
coconut butter
walnuts

DIRECTIONS:

01   Cut melon in half, remove seeds. Slice into 1 inch thick half moon slices using one of the halves of the melon. Cut rind off each half moon slice and proceed to cut into brownie sized squares.

02   Smear coconut butter on each santa claus melon square.

03   Top each piece with half a walnut.

Enjoy! :)

Note: If you can't find santa claus melon, honeydew melon can be used in its place.

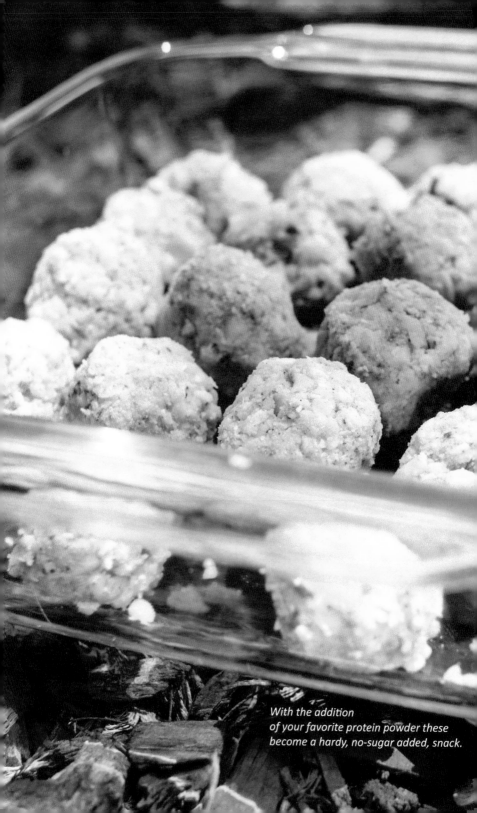

With the addition
of your favorite protein powder these
become a hardy, no-sugar added, snack.

COCONUT MAC BALLS

SERVES 8-10

INGREDIENTS:

1 cup macadamia nuts
1/3 cup cashews
1/3 cup walnuts
1/4 cup coconut butter
1/4 cup almond butter
1/3 cup unsweetened shredded coconut
1 tablespoon cinnamon
2 tablespoons coconut oil
2 tablespoons protein powder, *optional*

DIRECTIONS:

01 Add the macadamia nuts, cashews and walnuts to a food processor and run for a little over a minute or until you have medium sized chunks. Don't blend too long otherwise you'll have nut butter.

02 Add nut mixture to a medium sized bowl. Then add remaining ingredients.

03 Mix together until fully combined.

04 Scoop about 1 tablespoon of the mixture into your hands and roll into a ball.

05 Add to a glass dish, cover and store in the refrigerator.

Enjoy! :)

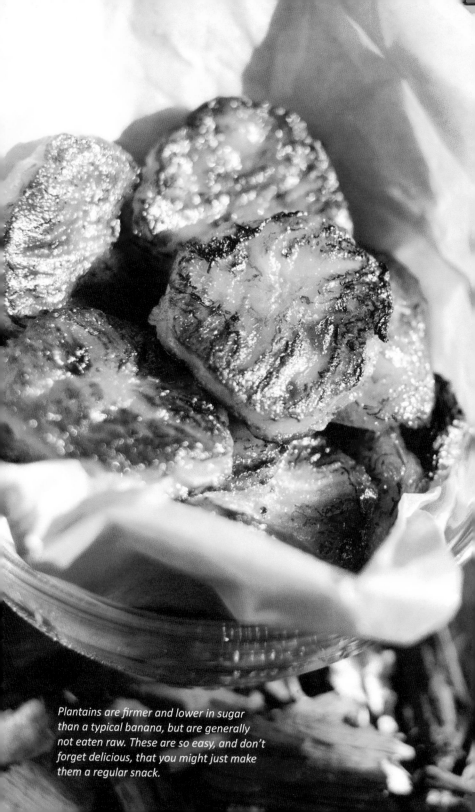

Plantains are firmer and lower in sugar than a typical banana, but are generally not eaten raw. These are so easy, and don't forget delicious, that you might just make them a regular snack.

COCONUT SEARED PLANTAINS

SERVES 4

INGREDIENTS:

2 plantains, sliced
coconut oil

DIRECTIONS:

01   Melt coconut oil in frying pan over medium high heat.

02   Cover the bottom of the frying pan with the sliced plantains, don't walk away. Watch to make sure they don't burn. After a minute or two give them a flip. You want them to get slightly browned but not charred and there's a fine line between when they turn.

03   Empty the first round of plantains onto a plate and feel free to pop one or two right in your mouth (but be warned they're hot, don't burn yourself).

04   Add more coconut oil to the pan, if needed, and refill with the second round of sliced plantains.

05   Repeat steps 3-4 until you've cooked all your plantains.

Enjoy! :)

For more recipes and a regular dose of Paleo Porn
visit me at MARLAsarris.com

A very special thank you goes out to Jeff Sarris, Dave LaTulippe, Vic Magary, Joel Runyon, Adam King, Bob and Michelle Gammelgaard, Joshua Fields Millburn, Ryan Nicodemus, Heather Allard, Ed, Gina, Amanda and Hannah Ceaser, Chris and Teri Sarris and everyone else who's supported and encouraged me throughout the years. This book would not have been possible without each and every one of you. Thank you all so much.